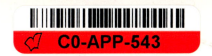

A
Principle
with
Promise

A Principle with Promise

Bert L. Fairbanks

*Eating and Exercising
Your Way to Health*

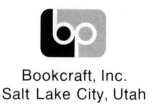

Bookcraft, Inc.
Salt Lake City, Utah

Library of Congress Catalog Card Number: 78-55416
ISBN 0-88494-340-2

First Printing, 1978

Lithographed in the United States of America
PUBLISHERS PRESS
Salt Lake City, Utah

To Gerri –
also to Tracy, Lori,
Becky, and Stephanie

Contents

Preface

Ever since the Prophet Joseph Smith received the Word of Wisdom (D&C 89), the world's science has been catching up. Latter-day Saints are familiar with the many findings of scientists concerning the harmful effects of tobacco, alcohol, and coffee and tea. But what many Saints aren't aware of is the fact that research in the fields of medicine and nutrition has also supported the rest of the Word of Wisdom — the suggestions about grains, about "every herb in the season thereof, and every fruit in the season thereof," about using meat "sparingly, . . . only in times of winter, or of cold, or famine." (D&C 89:11-13.)

These aspects of the Word of Wisdom are not viewed as commandments by the Church — but they are still the Lord's advice as to how we should take care of the bodies he has given us. By many standards, Latter-day Saints are the healthiest of all Americans. If we have received that blessing simply because we abstain from tobacco, alcohol, coffee, and tea, how much healthier we could be if we obeyed the entire Word of Wisdom!

Nutritional science is still in its infancy. Many things remain to be learned. But it is hardly surprising that as more is discovered about the body's requirements for food and exercise, the Word of Wisdom is continually found to be leading the way. Latter-day Saints can, today, keep their bodies in perfect condition by following the nutritional counsel which the Lord revealed for "the temporal salvation of all saints in the last days." (D&C 89:2.)

1

A Law
Anyone Can Live

The Word of Wisdom is one of the best-known aspects of the gospel. Ask a nonmember of the Church what he knows about the Mormons, and chances are pretty good that if he knows anything at all, he knows that Mormons don't drink alcohol, coffee, or tea, and that Mormons don't smoke.

But it's important for Saints to realize that the Word of Wisdom is more than a list of *don'ts*. It's like the law of the Sabbath: if you concentrate on all the things that aren't allowed on the Sabbath, you can easily begin to feel very deprived, and the day can be one that you dread. But the Lord would rather we concentrate on the positive that day — "Remember the sabbath day," he said, "to keep it holy." And when we think of all the good things that *can* and *should* be done on the Sabbath, things that we can't do during the week because we simply don't have time, then the day becomes one to be longed for, a day of rejoicing.

The Word of Wisdom is also a positive commandment, not a negative one. The Lord has not just hemmed us about with restrictions. Instead, he has pointed out the right way for us to treat our bodies. His guidelines are broad, and easily fol-

lowed. In fact, he said that the Word of Wisdom was "adapted
to the capacity of the weak and the weakest of all saints, who
are or can be called saints." (D&C 89:3.)

Imagine! A nutritional law adapted to the weakest among
us! The Lord gave us an easy law to follow; and yet how many
of us even know what the rest of the Word of Wisdom says,
let alone follow it?

"The letter killeth, but the spirit giveth life," said Paul to
the Corinthians — and to us, nearly two thousand years later.
(2 Cor. 3:6.) Right now, the Church only requires that its
members abstain from tobacco, alcohol, tea, and coffee — the
rest of the Word of Wisdom is voluntary. But just because the
Church has not strictly required that the Saints follow that law
to the letter does not mean that they should not try to follow
the spirit of the Word of Wisdom. "He that doeth not anything until he is commanded, and receiveth a commandment
with doubtful heart, and keepeth it with slothfulness, the
same is damned.... For behold, it is not meet that I should
command in all things; for he that is compelled in all things,
the same is a slothful and not a wise servant." (D&C 58:26,
29.)

But it is not just a question of obedience. Intelligent self-
interest should also lead the Lord's children to heed his advice
to them. The Lord called the Word of Wisdom "a principle
with promise," and told his prophet that "all saints who
remember to keep and do these sayings ... shall receive
health in their navel and marrow in their bones."

Do you feel sluggish, torpid, unable to think well because
your body is weary or hovering on the edge of illness? If you
obey the complete Word of Wisdom, the Lord has promised
that you "shall find wisdom and great treasures of knowledge, even hidden treasures."

Do you avoid climbing stairs or running to catch a bus
because you know it will wear you out too quickly? Do you
find yourself panting after the slightest unusual exertion? If
you "keep and do these sayings," the Lord has said that you
"shall run and not be weary."

And when you have to carry on even a mild exercise for a

long time, do you find that you simply haven't the endurance to walk just a few miles without stopping frequently to rest? Even carrying a bulky package, do you find that you have to keep changing positions because your arms haven't the endurance to hold it for very long? The Lord has promised that if you walk "in obedience to the commandments," you "shall walk and not faint."

And in perhaps the greatest promise of all, the Lord says that even beyond all these earthly rewards, obedience can lead you to the greatest reward of all. "And I, the Lord, give unto them a promise, that the destroying angel shall pass by them, as the children of Israel, and not slay them." (D&C 89:18-21.)

Americans — and citizens of other industrialized countries — have more food available to them than any other people in the history of the world. And yet we still manage to be undernourished; we still manage to take harmful substances into our bodies with practically every mouthful; we still mistreat our marvelous bodies, keeping them from working at their greatest potential.

Why?

Up to the time of the Word of Wisdom in 1833, people didn't have the ability to alter nature's foods that we have today. Your bread was baked from wheat you grew yourself — or purchased from a neighbor. You could see, if you wanted, the chicken that laid the eggs you ate, the cow that gave the milk you made into butter and cheese, the field where your beans and turnips grew, the tree from which your apples and peaches were picked.

But as people moved from the farm into the city and its suburbs, mass preparation and marketing of foods came into being. It was impossible for many years to bring fresh foods the required distances from field to table — and so canning, drying, salting, and other methods of preserving food were developed.

And then we began to find ways to refine foods, making them smoother, milder, sweeter — and, far too often, less nutritional. Our tastes changed, and instead of wanting bet-

ter, healthier foods, we began to want *faster* foods — faster to
prepare, faster to eat — and sweeter foods, piling on sugar
until the original flavor of the ingredients was lost.

For centuries, meat had been a luxury of the rich. Turkey,
ham, or goose became traditional at Christmas because that
was often the only time of the year when a poor or even
middle-class family might have that much meat. But as modern people became more prosperous, they began to buy more
of the meat that had so long been kept from them. And from
deprivation we turned to glut: today there are fewer families
than ever before who feel that a meal without meat is
adequate.

Why do we eat meat today as if we were starved for it?
Why do we insist on highly refined, oversweetened food at
every meal — and between? Why do we rely on instant,
ready-to-eat, just-add-water meals in our homes; and why do
we frequent fast-food restaurants where we can get a meal
from the grill to the table in five minutes, without regard to
nutrition?

"Behold, verily, thus saith the Lord unto you: In consequence of evils and designs which do and will exist in the
hearts of conspiring men in the last days, I have warned you,
and forewarn you, by giving unto you this word of wisdom by
revelation." (D&C 89:4.)

I seriously doubt that very many company executives sit
down together and say, "Well, let's see — how can we best
malnourish the American public *this* year?" But unfortunately, they have found that overrefined, improper foods often
sell much better than health-promoting foods. And because
their first obligation is to their stockholders, and not to the
purchasing public, they produce food products that will sell
better, often with little regard to nutritional value.

What they don't realize is that their stockholders eat, too!

We all eat. But *what* we eat makes a great deal of difference
in our lives. Improper foods can keep us alive for years, just as
smoking doesn't cause lung cancer the first week a person
smokes. But improper foods don't allow us to be truly
healthy.

After all, health isn't just the state of not being ill. Health is the ability to use the body to perform all needful activities; health is strength, vigor, endurance, and a robust appearance; health is lack of fatigue, the ability to think and make decisions quickly, unhampered by physical lethargy; health is bringing the body to the same level of perfection to which the Lord admonishes us to bring our spirits. "The spirit and the body are the soul of man," said the Lord, and it is our resurrected soul that we will keep through eternity — a good reason for using both body and spirit wisely and well. (D&C 88:15-16.)

Health isn't to be found in a doctor's office. Physicians freely admit that people only come to them when their bodies have begun malfunctioning so badly that they can no longer carry out their normal activity. But before body malfunctions reach that point, a steady, long-range pattern of deterioration can continue, virtually unnoticed, for years.

Without feeling the least bit ill, the human body, composed as it is of millions of body cells performing many different functions, can still be in poor health. But by following in detail the general guidelines in the Word of Wisdom, people can keep all their body cells, every tissue, every organ, functioning properly. In the final analysis, the health of human beings depends to a great extent upon the farmers who grow our food, the middlemen who prepare it and package it and market it, and the cooks who finally bring it to our tables.

However, health can't be divided into neat little packages. Though the body is made of many separate elements, they cannot be nourished and cared for separately. Individual cells are "alive" in the sense that they can reproduce and absorb and use up energy — but without the rest of the body to sustain them, cells cannot survive. We can't possibly nourish one portion of our body without some effect on all the other parts. And when we malnourish one part of our body, the rest of our being suffers, too.

Poor health, then, can't be remedied by one small change here and there, though indeed there are some changes that *can* make a dramatic difference. Total health comes from a totally healthy way of life, including the way we eat, the way we use our bodies, and the way we deal with the Lord and our fellowmen.

A complete different lifestyle? But how can a person change, when he has to live in the world?

Admittedly, it would be much easier if we could all travel to some city, a Zion where only pure foods were available to eat, where every person would be encouraged by the social system to get plenty of exercise, where the Spirit of God permeated every activity, every word, every thought. But remember — such a Zion has existed several times on the earth. And each time, it was made by ordinary people who lived in the world, but who were converted to the gospel and who completely changed their lives to fit the Lord's pattern.

What was the result for them? Happiness, health, strength, peace — and while many things in the world seem out of our control, surely one thing we can each control is what we take into our bodies and how we treat our bodies!

Because of the Word of Wisdom, there are several common misconceptions that Latter-day Saints should *not* have:

1. *The complete Word of Wisdom is nearly impossible to live.* Actually, it has never been easier to follow the Word of Wisdom than it is today. Centuries ago, people could only eat foods grown nearby, and while that food was healthful, they couldn't have much variety in their diets. Today, however, fresh, wholesome food can be purchased that was grown far from our supermarkets. All we have to do is be careful, not necessarily choosing the fastest and easiest way to eat, but instead choosing the most nutritive. After all, the Lord said the Word of Wisdom was adapted to the capacity of the weakest of the Saints!

2. *You can trust a brand-name that advertises heavily.* Too often we buy food because we have seen it advertised. When we do, we are forgetting the Lord's warning about "evil and conspiring men." Though some advertised foods may indeed be all they claim, many are not; and many are downright harmful.

3. *As long as it isn't alcohol, tobacco, coffee, or tea, it's all right.* Cyanide isn't mentioned in the Word of Wisdom, either, but there are few Latter-day Saints rushing out to get a good dose

— and yet we unwittingly (or wittingly!) take many poisons into our bodies in everyday foods. Colas aren't the only soft drinks that contain caffeine. And other substances in common preservatives or supplements added to processed foods can, over the years, have definite debilitating effects.

4. *There's a pill for every ill.* About fifteen tons of aspirin (acetylsalicylic acid) are consumed every day in the United States. People take aspirin so often that one might suppose a headache is the result of *not* having enough aspirin in the system! What many people don't realize is that most medicines are less effective the more we use them. If we take aspirin often, then when a really severe pain comes along, a much more powerful pain reliever must be used to contain it.

Likewise, many cold remedies, sleeping pills, and tranquilizers have side effects that we simply don't want! And most home remedy drugs relieve only the symptoms — they cure nothing at all. So while we go blissfully along with a nasal decongestant, two aspirin, and a mild tranquilizer calming our nerves, we can be seriously unhealthy, with nothing being done about it at all!

5. *Protein comes from meat.* Protein comes from wheat, too, and beans, and eggs and milk, and in small amounts from many other foods. The proteins in meat can be obtained elsewhere, and though we are counseled that meat is a proper food for man, the Lord has said, "It is pleasing unto me that [meat] should not be used, only in times of winter, or of cold, or famine." (D&C 89:13.) Latter-day Saints should be aware that when Joseph Smith recorded this revelation, the word *only* was used the way we use the word *except* today. Reading the scripture with that in mind removes any possible confusion about the Lord's intended meaning.

6. *Energy comes from sugar.* Actually, energy can also come from starches, fats, and proteins. Anyone who has ever compared the number of calories in a steak and the number in a bowl of spaghetti can testify that there is plenty of energy in unsugared foods, since a calorie *is* a unit for measuring energy. The true statement about sugar is that it provides *nothing* but energy. While the human body needs several thousand calories of energy a day to stay alive, it also needs dozens of

other nutrients; if a person's energy needs were met with nothing but pure sugar, it contains so little else that he would die of malnutrition — starving to death on thousands of calories a day! And foods that rely heavily on sugar, like candy, cakes, and many quick snack foods, provide little more than pure sugar.

7. *If I eat right and exercise, I'll be healthy.* You'll be healthier than those who don't, of course, but the Word of Wisdom has left nothing to chance. The promises from the Lord are extended to "all saints who remember to keep and do these sayings, *walking in obedience to the commandments.*" (D&C 89:18; emphasis added.) You can't be healthy if you're in turmoil because of arguments with people close to you. You can't be healthy if you work such a frenetic schedule that you don't get enough good sleep. You can't be healthy if you are so worried about worldly problems that you are constantly tense.

To be completely healthy, your whole life must be tuned to the Lord's pattern, both temporally and spiritually.

In a revelation received only two months before the Word of Wisdom, Joseph Smith recorded the Lord's instructions to the Saints: "Cease to be idle; cease to be unclean; cease to find fault one with another; cease to sleep longer than is needful; retire to thy bed early, that ye may not be weary; arise early, that your bodies and your minds may be invigorated.

"And above all things, clothe yourselves with the bond of charity, as with a mantle, which is the bond of perfectness and peace." (D&C 88:124-25.)

The gospel does not teach us to be exclusively spiritual, neglecting our bodies. It teaches us to prepare our whole soul, body and spirit, to dwell with the Lord.

Often people go through life seeing nothing good or enjoyable in their physical make-up, finding themselves too short, too tall, their nose too large, their eyes too close together. And while they mourn the things about their body that they can't change, they neglect those aspects that they can change, letting themselves become weak, fatigued, obese, undernourished and overfed. They are dissatisfied with their bodies because they have never learned to treat them and use them properly. They have never experienced the harmonious relationship of mind and body striving toward a common goal.

To enjoy the full benefits of the Word of Wisdom, we must incorporate into our lives the pure love of Christ; we must clothe ourselves "with the bond of charity, as with a mantle." Nobody can be healthy *alone.* The peace and happiness that allow complete health to reign can only come when we have deep and harmonious relationships with other children of our Father. The gospel relieves the insecurity of the lonely soul by linking us tightly to family, forever; it eases the anxiety of the searching soul by answering the profoundest questions of life; it eliminates idleness by providing constant opportunity to serve our fellowmen, both within the Church and outside it; and it cancels fear, by letting us come to know God, love the Savior, and become constant companions with the Holy Spirit.

I

Eating Intelligently

"How strange a creature is man, who will at times go to such extremes to preserve his life, only to shorten it at the dinner table."

—William H. Gordon

2

Something
Is Very Wrong

In 1973, the results of a nationwide survey of Canadians were announced. An alarming number of people suffered from overweight, undernutrition, and anemia. Iron deficiencies were especially pronounced among women of childbearing years. Many Canadians of all ages suffered from deficiencies of folic acid, a B vitamin that aids in the proper transfer of heredity characteristics from a body cell to the next generation as it reproduces within the body.

And it isn't just Canada! The U.S. Department of Agriculture discovered in 1965 that since 1955 the nutritional quality of Americans' diets had fallen remarkably — even though Americans were becoming more prosperous and better able to buy good food. The nutrients Americans were most likely to be lacking were calcium, vitamin A, and ascorbic acid — vitamin C. And things haven't improved since then. A national expenditure of billions of dollars on medical care hints that all is not well with the nation's health. In fact, in 1972 the Department of Agriculture "speculated that good eating habits could cut the incidence of heart and vascular diseases by 25%, reduce respiratory infections by 20% and slash arthritis, diabetes and infant mortality by half.'' (*Time Magazine,* December 18, 1972.)

What? The number-one killer of Americans, heart disease, could be cut by one-fourth if people would only eat properly? Well, as soon as Americans know *that* you can be sure they'll change their eating habits and save their lives!

But that was 1972, and today we're eating as badly as ever — if not worse.

Medicine isn't enough to give you good health. Even preventive medicine is like trying to win a football game by keeping the other team from scoring. At best, you can only come up with a tie — zero to zero. In order to win the reward of total health, you have to score. You have to have a positive approach to nutrition and body care that will make you so strong that only the most powerful of diseases can strike you; so strong that even when you are ill, your body can fend off the disease quickly; so strong that when you have to make exceptional demands on your body, your body is able to respond.

Where does malnutrition begin?

In the womb.

The developing embryo and, later, fetus depend on the mother for every nutrient they receive. Eighty percent of all brain growth occurs between the moment of conception and the age of two — and if, during those crucial years, the unborn child or the infant are undernourished, the growth lost then can never be made up.

And how quickly children learn the patterns of malnutrition! The reward for good behavior or the special family treat is rarely a carrot or a glass of milk — it's a candy bar or an ice cream cone. The quick snack with friends is never celery or a hard-boiled egg — it's a soft drink or a bag of barbecue-flavored potato chips.

There's no time for lunch— and so we stop at a fast food restaurant and stock up on empty calories.

We've got no way to prepare proper meals while we're traveling — and so on vacation the family snacks its way to a week of malnutrition.

No wonder that one writer on the subject of nutrition titled his article, "We Feed Our Hogs Better Than Our Children"! (*American Magazine,* October 1947.) After all, farmers watch carefully every aspect of their livestock's diet. An improperly fed hog or steer brings a lower market price; an improperly fed and cared for chicken doesn't lay enough eggs.

But children often grow up hardly knowing a brussels sprout from broccoli, because they haven't eaten either of them often enough to remember what they're called. Yet those same children can tell you the difference between a quarter-pounder and a superburger, between diet soft drinks and the regular kind, between one candy bar and its closest rival.

We make far too many of our eating choices out of habit. Accustomed to eating sugar, we want more sugar; addicted to chocolate, we crave ever larger quantities; tied to social customs that insist on soft drinks (or hard drinks!), we hardly dare insist on something healthier.

"What? Tomato juice with a hamburger?"

Well, you could skip the hamburger, too, and eat something healthier.

"Forget it. I like hamburgers."

But why do you like hamburgers? Because you're used to them, along with cake for dessert, cookies for treats, and catsup with french fries. With a little effort you could get used to something better for you, something that could help you live longer, something that could make your life more enjoyable as you live through it.

"But it doesn't *taste* like a hamburger!"

It will surprise you how quickly you'll come to enjoy a different way of eating. And as many people who have cut down on harmful or empty foods have discovered, after only a few weeks of proper eating, those "favorite foods" of a few weeks ago don't taste very good at all. It doesn't take long to learn to prefer good food to bad.

How can you tell if you're undernourished?

1. If you're substantially over or under the normal weight for your height, body frame, and age, or if, during the growing years, you just aren't growing.

2. If you have poor posture; if your chest protrudes, your

shoulders are rounded, your abdomen is thrust forward, your back is swayed.

3. If your muscles are thin and flabby; if you seem to have no padding of fat, or far too much.

4. If your skin is dry, scaly, and pale, and you have pale mucous membranes.

5. If your jaw is poorly formed with teeth poorly aligned.

6. If your hair is dull and dry.

7. If your eyes are dull or oversensitive to light; if they often burn or itch; if you have circles or puffiness under your eyes.

8. If you have a poor appetite, or often complain of indigestion, and if you crave sweets and highly seasoned foods.

9. If you are listless, easily fatigued, and have little endurance.

10. If you are prone to become ill often, or if illnesses keep you abed longer than normal.

11. If you have a short attention span and just can't seem to concentrate.

12. If you're irritable, apathetic, worried, or depressed much of the time.

13. If you often can't sleep well, or if you awaken feeling tired and out of sorts.

Of course, some of these are not always signs of poor nutrition. But a significant number of them are a fairly certain indicator that something is wrong with your diet.

Look at your children, your parents, your husband or wife, and see if they seem to be getting proper nourishment. And ask them if you show these symptoms, too. The answer may surprise you.

And if you and your family *are* undernourished, are you willing to change? It will mean a great deal of care at first, as you establish new routines and patterns. The day may have to be scheduled more carefully to be certain there are no mad dashes to the store for instant, empty meals. The shopping list will probably have to be thrown away and a new one developed. And whoever prepares the food will have to learn new methods, new menus, and new patience to endure the inevitable complaints as the family begins to adjust.

Does it sound like a lot of bother? After all, the only thing you get in return is a 25 percent lower chance of heart disease, half the chance of diabetes, strength and endurance that will surprise you, far greater happiness, and more energy to live the kind of life you always wanted to.

There are two extremes to avoid in eating habits. The most common is the unthinking selection of food for taste and preference alone, with no concern for nutrition; the other is the fanatical overconcern of the food faddist. In both cases, life is revolving around the diet, instead of the diet being shaped to promote a good life. And food faddists become easy prey to food quacks who promise health from eating certain special foods or nutritional supplements. Advertisements are aimed at your pocketbook, not at your health, whether the pitchman is shouting "Dinner in a minute" or "Health in a week."

Health doesn't come from "magic" foods or clever-looking capsules. Health is the direct but not always instantaneous result of obedience to the natural laws which lead to an abundant and full life.

You're surrounded by abundance; supermarkets contain a constantly bountiful harvest from millions of well-tended acres. But chances are that you're undernourished, starved for certain vital nutrients. And all the while, you're gorging yourself on hundreds of empty, unhelpful calories.

Something is very wrong.

You eat, and eat again, and yet you're still hungry.

3

The Grain,
the Whole Grain, and
Nothing but the Grain

I have been taught for years that wheat and the other grains, while they were rich in protein and carbohydrates, did not contain "complete proteins." The theory was that some vital proteins had to be obtained from meat.

And then it occurred to me to wonder how in the world cows and hogs and chickens got *their* "complete proteins." After all, they live entirely on grains and other vegetable products.

If these animals can get complete proteins from a vegetarian diet, why can't human beings?

Obviously, some information was missing. Or perhaps I had been taught incorrectly for years, and grains *do* contain those complete proteins.

What are proteins? Essentially, they are the building blocks of life — all life, from viruses to plants to people. Composed of relatively simple molecules called amino acids, proteins are present in every living cell.

There are twenty-two amino acids known to be commonly present in proteins. And yet these twenty-two components of proteins, like the twenty-six letters of the alphabet, can be combined and recombined in a virtually uncountable array of combinations. And each different combination is a different type of protein, fitted to do a different kind of job within the body.

If we think of amino acids as letters, and proteins as the words made from them, then the "vocabulary" of the human body ranges from little eight-letter words (proteins made of eight amino acids) to long eighteen-letter words — real jaw-breakers! And just as the word *strength* is different from the word *conceptualization*, the different words in our protein vocabulary do completely different jobs. The proteins in our teeth, bones, or fingernails are thoroughly different from the proteins in muscle tissue or in the liver.

When we eat, almost all our food will contain at least some protein (though in some cases the protein is negligible). However, our body can't use most protein in the form in which it occurs in our food. After all, we don't need many plant proteins in our bodies, and when we eat beef we don't hope the protein will simply add bovine muscles to our bodies — we need *human* proteins.

So during digestion, our bodies break down proteins into the amino acids they were made of. A protein "word" (like *beefsteak*) gets broken down into its nine letters, or individual amino acids. Then our bodies recombine these amino acids in the individual cells, turning them into the proteins we need — just as if we had scrambled up all the letters and chosen our own words from them.

Our bodies can even take the individual atoms that make up the amino acid molecules and recombine them into new amino acids. However, we can only do this with *some* amino acids — others have to come in the food we eat.

This is where "complete" and "incomplete" proteins come in. When a particular food contains the essential amino acids that our own bodies can't manufacture — and has them in roughly the proportions that our bodies need — then that food is said to provide complete proteins. Hen's eggs are the best source of complete proteins; other excellent sources are milk, cheese, fish, meat, and poultry.

Obviously, then, we have to eat meat — right? That's what

I was taught for many years. But let's take another look at the incomplete proteins. There isn't one single amino acid missing from one vegetable source that can't be found in another — there is no "letter" in our amino acid alphabet that can only be found in meat!

The amino acids that our body cannot make are:
Histidine (needed primarily by infants and children)
Isoleucine
Leucine
Lysine
Methionine
Phenylalanine
Threonine
Tryptophan
Valine

These are the essential amino acids, the ones that must be in our food, since our body can't manufacture them. And while meat provides all of them, combinations of various plant foods can equal the protein value of meat. For instance, corn alone is deficient, and so are dry beans. But when these two foods are eaten at the same meal — a common Latin American combination — all the essential proteins are provided.

Wheat is almost complete. Its only deficiency is in lysine — and even that amino acid is not completely missing. In fact, wheat is so complete that only 1.5 cups of wheat per day would meet all the amino acid requirements of the human body — including lysine!

However, the process of refining wheat into white flour — the most common way we eat wheat today — removes much of the lysine, wheat's weak point. A much greater amount of refined white flour is necessary in order to meet the body's needs.

When you buy white flour, chances are that on the package the word *enriched* is prominently displayed. That means that some nutrients have been added to the white flour — nutrients which were in the whole wheat originally, but which were stripped out during the refining process.

However, not all the lost nutrients are restored when the white flour is "enriched." One important nutrient that is lost during the refining of flour is vitamin E.

Though vitamin E has been known for years, it remained a mystery — no one was sure what it actually did. Many even believed that it wasn't essential to the human body. But Franklin Bicknell wrote as long ago as 1953, "It is fantastic to believe that while mice and monkeys, ducks and dogs, beetles and barrows all need vitamin E, yet a beneficent and wise biological providence has excused man from this irksome necessity.

"It is impossible to believe that vitamin E is not essential for men, but it well may be that the symptoms of prolonged mild deficiency only show themselves after many years, and then are so blurred by the changes of sensibility which they themselves help to produce, that they are difficult, or even impossible, to recognize. It is grievous that our food loses so much of what may be an essential protection against senility merely because the vision of science is just as long as the life of a rat." (Bicknell and Prescott, *The Vitamins in Medicine*, New York: Grune and Straton, 1953.)

Today the function of vitamin E in man is beginning to be understood — and its almost complete lack in our diet is more than a little frightening. Doctors graduating from medical school as recently as 1911 had never heard of coronary thrombosis. Yet today that condition has reached epidemic proportions in the United States, Canada, and other industrialized countries. It is now responsible for more than 50 percent of all deaths. An ever-increasing number of young men are being struck down before the age of forty, at a time when they are most needed by their families and when they are prepared to make their greatest contribution to society.

Why has coronary thrombosis become so common in only the last few years? Many explanations have been suggested — stress and strain, overexertion, the fast pace of modern living, soft drinking water (or hard drinking water), and of course diets rich in saturated fats. Each explanation has some plausibility — until you realize that every single one of those conditions could be found before the twentieth century. Why, then, have heart attacks become epidemic today?

A coronary thrombosis occurs when a blood clot develops in one of the tiny arteries that feed blood to the heart (the heart, like any other muscle, needs blood to stay alive, and the blood pumping through the chambers of the heart doesn't reach the strong outer muscle, where most of the work of the circulatory system is done). When that blood clot stays lodged in the artery where it formed, it is called a thrombus. Eventually, more and more blood clots with the thrombus, until no more blood can flow through the artery past that point.

If the blocked artery is not a particularly important one, other blood vessels can often make up the slack, and the coronary thrombosis is barely noticed. However, when the thrombus blocks the blood supply to a large area of the heart, the heart simply stops beating — and the victim has a heart attack.

Why do those little blood clots form? It has been widely held that the cause was atherosclerosis — build-ups of deposits on the insides of the arteries, which make them narrower and therefore easier to block. But while atherosclerosis certainly doesn't help, it also isn't the primary cause of coronary thrombosis. Many heart attacks occur when there is no atherosclerosis.

Recent studies are linking coronary thrombosis with vitamin E deficiency. Vitamin E has been found not only to help dissolve clots in the bloodstream, but also, when it is circulating normally through the blood, to keep those clots from forming at all. And with vitamin E keeping the blood flowing smoothly, even serious atherosclerosis does not necessarily result in a heart attack. (See Wilfrid E. Shute, *Vitamin E for Ailing and Healthy Hearts,* Pyramid, 1972.)

When new and more efficient milling methods were introduced into the manufacture of wheat flour at the turn of the century, for the first time the wheat germ was completely stripped from the grain — and the flour became totally white. With this process, the diet of western man lost its only significant source of vitamin E. Since 1910, when this refining process first became general, and today — when 98 percent of wheat consumed is in the form of highly refined white flour, coronary thrombosis has increased until more than a million people die of it each year in the United States alone.

And vitamin E is not the only nutrient lost in the refining of white flour. Vitamin B-6 (pyridoxin) is also removed, with no attempt made to restore it. And even some of the nutrients added to "enriched" white flour are not as effective as the same nutrients in unstripped whole wheat.

For instance, a research team at the Utah State University discovered that the iron added to "enriched" white flour is not as easily absorbed by the body as iron naturally occurring in wheat. Fourteen percent of the iron in enriched white bread was utilized by experimental animals — while 27 percent of the iron in whole wheat flour was usable.

Why is there a difference? Iron is iron, isn't it?

If iron were iron, no matter what form it was in, we could go to the mines for our dietary iron! But iron is used by the body as part of various compounds — iron atoms combined with other atoms to make more complex molecules. These iron atoms, vital to form compounds in the body — particularly in the blood, where iron is part of our oxygen-carrying system — can more easily be extracted from some compounds than from others. And the whole grain wheat carries iron in a much more accessible form than "enriched" white flour.

Of course, not all refining of modern foods is harmful. Thousands of people used to die every year from contaminants in natural milk, until pasteurization became the almost universal method of purifying milk so that it no longer carried disease. But often refining disturbs chemical balances that are at first unnoticed. For years we have believed that vitamin C is vitamin C, regardless of whether it occurs naturally or is chemically processed ascorbic acid. But in 1974 chromatography research revealed that the intricate patterns produced in the body by naturally occurring vitamin C are due, in part, to biologically active ingredients that accompany the vitamin C, some of which are proteins and enzymes. Synthetic vitamin C contains no such proteins and enzymes, since these are all removed during the refining process. And other nutrients can be harmed or their efficiency reduced because of BHA and BHT, the most common commercial food preservatives. (*Prevention Magazine,* January 1974.)

It has been suggested that overrefined carbohydrates, which predominate in our diet, may well contribute to cancer of the colon, which is emerging as a leading cause of death in industrialized nations.

If whole wheat flour is so much more nutritive than refined white flour, why do we consume 98 percent of the wheat we eat in the form of white flour? The most common reasons are:

1. *White flour can be stored indefinitely.* Whole wheat flour must be used within relatively narrow limits of time, while white flour doesn't spoil as easily. For this reason, commerce requires white flour, so that it can be stored and shipped over long distances. A possible solution of this problem might be the decentralization of flour mills, so that those long distances can be eliminated.

It has been facetiously suggested that the main reason white flour stores so much better than whole wheat flour is that so many nutrients have been removed that the bacteria and insects that make whole wheat flour spoil can't survive on white flour!

2. *It is not economical to decentralize flour milling.* This is true. Whole wheat flour would have to be ground in smaller amounts, more often, and closer to the markets. It would need to be refrigerated to prevent spoilage between the mill and the cities. All of this would increase the cost.

But it's cheaper than losing our health! How much money is our health worth to us? And will the stockholders of the refining companies earn enough in profits to make it worth increasing the risk of heart attacks, cancer, and other physiological disasters?

3. *White bread looks more pure.* Whiteness is often associated with purity. And in a sense, white bread *is* more pure. After all, so much has been removed from it! So far as contaminants are concerned, however, white bread is no more pure than whole wheat bread — and the missing nutrients make it far less valuable as food.

4. *People like the taste and texture of white flour foods.* But this is just the result of habit. People raised on whole wheat flour products find white flour products bland or weak. Given time, we would learn to like — and even prefer — the taste and texture of the more healthful whole wheat flour in our food.

5. *Whole wheat flour is too rough for the digestive system.* Properly ground, whole wheat flour is every bit as fine as white flour — it just contains the whole grain, instead of having only a part of the grain. And the higher fiber content of whole wheat flour actually improves digestion.

The Lord told us, "All grain is good for the food of man." But of all the grains, he said, "Nevertheless, wheat for man. . . ." (D&C 89:16-17.) Wheat is the staff of life — as long as we use the grain properly, and don't remove much of what makes it such a valuable source of the proteins, vitamins, minerals, and carbohydrates our bodies need.

4

Over-Meating

"Meat is the best source of protein," say many experts, and they're right. But that doesn't make meat the perfect food. If you knew that a juicy slice of ham, besides being full of protein, was also loaded down with trichina cysts ready to infest you with worms, how tempted would you be to eat it?

It's not enough just to know that meat is full of protein. In order to understand the role it should play in our diet, we need to know *everything*, good and bad, that meat provides.

Sometimes it seems there are only two positions on the use of meat. One is that meat is essential in the daily diet of every healthy person — and that the more meat you eat, the better off you are. The other is that meat is absolutely harmful, and shouldn't be eaten at all.

However, there is a middle ground — and that middle ground is where the Lord's word on the question stands. "And whoso forbiddeth to abstain from meats, that man should not eat the same, is not ordained of God," says the Lord, "for, behold, the beasts of the field and the fowls of the air, and that which cometh of the earth, is ordained for the use of man for food and for raiment, and that he might have in abundance." (D&C 49:18-19.)

So vegetarianism isn't part of the Lord's program. But neither is overuse of meat. "And wo be unto man that sheddeth blood or that wasteth flesh and hath no need." (D&C 49:21.) And when do we *have* a need? In the Word of Wisdom, the Lord urges, "Yea, flesh also of beasts and of the fowls of the air, I, the Lord, have ordained for the use of man with thanksgiving; nevertheless they are to be used sparingly;

"And it is pleasing unto me that they should not be used, only in times of winter, or of cold, or famine." (D&C 89:12-13.)

Furthermore, meat animals "hath God made for the use of man only in times of famine and excess of hunger." (D&C 89:15.)

It sounds like the Lord intends us to use meat only as an emergency food — a supplement when other, more proper foods are scarce or beyond our means to obtain them. Why? Why doesn't the Lord want us to take advantage of the abundance of meat and eat it constantly?

One reason may simply be disease. There are some one hundred diseases transmissible from animals to man. Often animals suffering from some of these diseases are consigned to a meat market, to be devoured as the entree on our supper tables. A 1969 U.S. Agriculture Department report said, "Today, based on the most recent incidence figures, between 80,000 and 90,000 trichina-infested hogs are marketed yearly." (Quoted in Owen S. Parrett, "Diseases of Food Animals," Washington, D.C.: 1974.)

Doesn't exactly make you want to reach for the bacon, does it?

Perhaps we should feel like Daniel, who refused to eat the king's meat. Test us for ten days, he asked the king, "and let them give us pulse [a porridge made of grains and legumes, like peas and beans], and water to drink. . . .

"And at the end of ten days their countenances appeared fairer and fatter in flesh than all the children which did eat the portion of the king's meat." (Dan. 1:12, 15.)

Daniel's experiment took place several thousand years ago — but a modern application of the same principle took place in Denmark during the First World War. Denmark imported most of its feed grain for cattle and hogs — and when the war blockades cut off the supply, four-fifths of the hogs and two-thirds of the dairy cattle were slaughtered. For a short time meat prices were ridiculously low, and the supply of meat was ample. But the situation quickly changed, and for several years the Danish diet consisted of "war bread" made from wheat and rye flour. Dr. Hindhede, the government's supervisor of the national diet, was in charge of creating a healthy diet that would fit well with rationing needs.

The diet eliminated alcoholic beverages; tea and coffee weren't available at all. Sugar was in short supply. Meat, butter, and milk were almost eliminated, and besides "war bread," only vegetables and a few fruits were available.

What happened to the Danes?

During the year of the involuntary experiment, the Danish death rate fell nearly one-fifth, and became the lowest ever known in Europe. In October 1918, when the influenza epidemic slaughtered huge numbers of Europeans — more than the war, in some countries — Denmark was the only noncombatant nation in Europe with a death rate during and after the disease *lower* than the death rate had been before the war began!

Elder and Sister John A. Widtsoe, the apostle, and his wife, Leah, commented on the Danish experience in their book *The Word of Wisdom:* "Abstinence from alcohol, tea and coffee, no doubt was a prime factor in reducing the normal death rate and in giving the nation resistance against the influenza scourge. In like manner a good diet of natural food will protect the body against most diseases today." (Deseret Book, 1950, p. 243.)

Meat is just not as necessary and helpful as many people have thought — and can cause definite harm. Even disease-free meat can be detrimental. Many products of meat digestion are distinctly acid, and can cause serious harm if excessive in quality. And since the waste products from meat are disposed of by the liver and kidneys, and not just by the intestines, excessive meat-eating can place undue strain on those organs. Also, excess of uric acid, a meat digestion by-product, and the putrefaction of proteins in the bowels often contribute to the development of such unpleasant conditions as gout, kidney stones, bladder stones, not to mention the much more common headaches, fatigue, and decreased resistance to disease that seem to be a constant plague in our modern society.

Pavlov, most famous for his experiments in conditioning behavior, also experimented with diet. He performed a delicate operation on a dog, sending blood directly from the small intestine, where food was digested and passed into the blood, to the heart. Normally, the blood would pass through the liver first. However, Pavlov bypassed that organ.

As long as the dog was fed on vegetable food, it lived on. When it was fed meat products, however, it quickly suffered convulsions and died.

There are poisons in meat — substances which act against the well-being of our bodies. In carnivorous animals, of course, very large livers cope easily with the poisons. But man has a relatively small liver. It just can't cope with the strain of a heavy meat diet.

Wait a minute — don't we have to have meat to be "big and strong"?

No — your body breaks meat proteins down into amino acids. Amino acids look alike, whether they come from vegetable or meat sources — but the extra poisons that meat brings can make a big difference. In fact, any scientific grounds for believing meat has something to do with strength disappeared long ago. In experiments conducted by Sparks, Roth, and Lewis, it was found that swimmers who abstained from meat entirely showed general improvement and had more stamina and endurance. Milk, much milder and less harmful, provided what proteins they didn't get from vegetables.

Much of the common belief that meat gives strength is sheer superstition. Just as cannibals often believed that by eating an enemy's brains they gained his wisdom, so we today believe that by eating the muscles of strong animals, we will gain their strength. However, *they* didn't gain that strength from eating meat!

Another strong argument in favor of cutting way down on meat consumption is simply that meat isn't a very economical way to eat. Cattle, hogs, and other meat animals have to eat grain to get their strength. But much of the caloric content of the vegetable feed they eat is used in keeping the animal alive — and that energy is never passed on to us. If we got the calories directly from vegetable products, instead of having them pass through meat animals first, we could get three to four times the nutrition — or, to put it another way, every time we eat a steak, we're really eating a plateful of vegetables, with three-fourths of the nutrition gone!

Can a whole society really be based on a diet that doesn't include much meat? There are many, today and in the past, that have done exactly that. For instance, the Hunzakuts, a people living near the northwest end of the Himalayas, have survived vigorously for centuries on a diet of grains, including wheat, barley, buckwheat, and small grains; leafy green vegetables; potatoes and other root vegetables; chick peas and other legumes (*pulses* — remember Daniel?); milk and buttermilk, clarified butter and cheese; fruit, particularly apricots and mulberries, both fresh and dried; and occasionally — *very* occasionally — meat.

What has it done for the Hunzakuts? They aren't a rich people, of course — except for that wealth that can't be bought with money: health. Men of ninety have been known to father children; women of fifty have been known to conceive and bear children. They haven't heard of the Word of Wisdom, of course, but as with all the Lord's blessings, the rewards of obedience come even when the obedience is entirely unwitting.

Another group with remarkably good results from a low-meat diet is found in Eastern Europe. The Bulgarians, in the 1930 census, were found to have 1,600 persons over 100 years of age out of every million persons in the country. The rate in the United States at the time was only nine centenarians per million. Furthermore, while few American centenarians are particularly spry, these old people in Bulgaria were still vigorous, still active — more like sixty-year-olds in America than like people of similar age.

What was the diet of Bulgarians at that time? Mostly black bread from whole rye flour and sour milk, or yogurt, made from ordinary milk soured by a microbe called the "Bulgarian bacillus." (Widtsoe, *Word of Wisdom*, p. 256.)

Immediately after World War II, thousands and thousands of Europeans were starving. Yet it was only after many weeks of deficient diet — deficient in everything, not just in meat — that a protein deficiency began to appear. And that protein deficiency was usually relieved just by giving them more of their normal diet: cereal grains and potatoes. "It is most unlikely," said those who reported that finding, "that protein deficiency will develop in apparently healthy adults on a diet in which cereals and vegetables supply adequate calories." (D. M. Hegsted, *Journal of Laboratory and Clinical Medicine* 31:261.)

One doctor discovered that when patients showed signs of kidney breakdown through the appearance of albumen and casts in the urine, the situation could be cleared up completely by putting them on a diet of fruits, vegetables, and salads, with all meat and even meat-based soups completely prohibited. And the kidney problems disappeared in only a week or two!

This is not to say, of course, that eating meat is going to kill you. The Lord is very clear on that point — meat is permissible, and at times desirable, for man. However, the Lord — and recent findings of science — make it clear that overuse of meat can and will do harm. Russell Henry Chittenden, a Yale physiological chemist, pointed out: "The smallest amount of food able to keep the body in a state of high efficiency is physiologically the most economical, and thus best adapted for the body's needs. Too little food is bad, but so is too much. The average American diet contains forty-five percent more protein than the National Academy of Sciences recommends: therefore, to that extent it is not 'best adapted to the body's needs.' " (Quoted in Raymond H. Woolsey, "Meat on the Menu: Who Needs It?" Review and Herald Publishing Association, 1974, p. 58.)

Perhaps it is not such a coincidence that as meat consumption in industrialized nations has increased dramatically, so
has the incidence of cancer. The late Dr. William J. Mayo of
the Mayo Clinic at Rochester, Minnesota, in an address before
the American College of Surgeons, cited the remarkable figure that American meat consumption has increased 400 percent in the last hundred years! And he went on to link this
with stomach cancer: "Cancer of the stomach forms nearly
one-third of all cancers of the human body. So far as I know,
this is not true of lower animals, nor of uncivilized man. It is
not possible, therefore, that there is something in the habits of
civilized man, in the cooking or other preparation of his food,
which acts to produce the precancerous condition? Within
the last one hundred years, four times as much meat is taken
as before that time. If flesh foods are not fully broken up,
decomposition results, and active poisons are thrown into an
organ not intended for their reception, and which has not had
time to adapt itself to the new condition."

That's serious business. Eating more meat than our bodies
can handle can eventually kill us! But the truth is that we've
been warned — for centuries. The Lord created human beings
in such a way that we can't cope with too large a quantity of
meat in our diet — and then warned us all amply that meat
should be avoided, except under certain conditions.

Nutritional science, while still in its infancy, has finally
overcome the myth that of the essential amino acids, all had to
be eaten in the right proportion in the same meal or the body
would immediately have a protein deficiency. Actually, the
body can go for some time without infusions of all the essential amino acids, by simply recycling those amino acids from
dead cells, digestive secretions, and so forth. The body is not
so fragile that a day without meat is a day of malnutrition. In
fact, the body makes its own balance of amino acids.

But while that myth had force, many doctors and many
athletic coaches insisted that the people they cared for eat
meat at every meal. And yet even if those essential amino
acids really did have to come from meat products, there
would be better ways to get them than muscle meat itself!

For example, eggs are a much more valuable source of

amino acids than muscle meat, largely because they are easier to digest fully and contain a higher percentage of available protein. They are also an excellent source of vitamin B-12, a nutrient that comes primarily from meat and meat products, though some current findings seem to indicate that B-12 can actually be synthesized by the human body when a good balance of fruits, vegetables, and legumes is eaten.

Another good source of animal protein is milk; and even the "organ meats" — liver, kidney, heart, and brain — are less harmful and more nutritive than muscle meats. And, of course, all the necessary proteins can just as easily be obtained from combinations of legumes (peas, beans, peanuts) and grain, or legumes and seeds, or grains and milk products.

As a matter of fact, it is much better to view meat the way the Lord wants us to — not as the basic food for which other foods are a substitute or a supplement, but rather as a substitute itself, to be eaten only when the more healthful combinations aren't available or aren't sufficient.

Eggs are a good protein source — but there are drawbacks. While they don't putrefy in the intestines quite as badly as muscle meat, they do putrefy. And eggs contain cholesterol, a substance thoroughly linked to atherosclerosis, the build-up of deposits on the walls of arteries, which can lead to strokes and heart attacks. However, very recently researchers have discovered that the amount of cholesterol a person *eats* has almost nothing to do with how the cholesterol is used in the body. In the experiments, blood cholesterol levels were measured for people who had eaten a large number of eggs, and for people who had avoided eggs and other cholesterol sources. It was found that there was no correlation between cholesterol build-up and the amount of cholesterol eaten. In fact, it was a chemical imbalance in the body that decided whether the extra cholesterol would be taken into the body or whether it would simply be flushed out at the earliest opportunity — and if that series of experiments is confirmed by more research, the days of fearing the cholesterol in eggs may be over!

Earlier tests seemed to point to this same result. Research on animals had already made it clear that egg yolks consumed in large quantities, all other things being equal, did not cause atherosclerosis. The real cause of atherosclerosis, it seems, is improper nutrition in the body cells — caused, in large measure, by the kind of general diet most Americans eat! Instead of cutting out eggs, victims of atherosclerosis should have kept the eggs — and got rid of the junk food, the empty calories, and the muscle meats!

Eggs are 74 percent water, with the other 26 percent fairly evenly divided between proteins and fats. Milk, too, is well-balanced, with 87 percent water, 3.5 percent protein, 3.9 percent fat, and 4.9 percent milk sugar. Also, 0.7 percent of milk is mineral matter, including calcium and phosphorus, greatly needed by the body for growth and repair. Milk also contains vitamins A, B-1, and B-2, and healthy doses of vitamin D. And the sugar in milk, lactose, is one of the few sugars that do not ferment, so that milk won't cause the digestive disturbance often caused by refined sugars.

Milk, like eggs, has been blamed for atherosclerosis — but instead of the fats in milk causing lesions and atherosclerosis, research has recently indicated that it is the *absence* of fats in milk that causes those conditions! A research team headed by Denizen found that nonfat dry milk caused atherosclerosis in rats, while milk with the butterfat intact did not. We may be hurting ourselves by removing the butterfat from milk.

And grains and vegetables, as discussed already, do not have the same balance of amino acids as meat — but in the right combinations, they provide everything needed for life. And a diet based on a good mixture of fruits, vegetables, legumes, and grains, supplemented by some milk and eggs, will certainly provide everything needed. Meat just isn't essential, and because it can cause harm, it should be avoided.

Rats aren't people — but they live faster than we do, and so the long-term results of certain diet patterns can be more easily seen in rats than in human populations. Besides, rats eat what they're fed! Dr. Mary Swartz Rose at Columbia University fed three groups of rats of the same age, size, and weight very different diets. Group A was allowed to eat as much as they wanted of pure whole wheat bread, whole milk, water, and a little salt. Group B was fed all they wanted of bread — and meat. And Group C got as much bread and eggs as they wanted.

Group A grew throughout forty-six generations with an ever-increasing degree of health, vigor, and power of reproduction. The last generation of rats were far healthier than the original group — their umpty-third great-grandparents who began the experiment. Group B, however, never got to forty-six generations. In fact, there was never a second generation. They lasted only a few weeks, and all died. Group C, fed with eggs and bread, fared just about as well as Group A.

Want a thick, rich, juicy steak?

How long do you want to live?

But wait a minute — weren't human beings *meant* to eat meat? Some writers have compared man's digestive system with the digestive system of herbivores and carnivores, and have concluded that there are more similarities to carnivores than to herbivores. This is partly explainable to Latter-day Saints by the fact that the Lord has told us that we *are* meant to eat meat — as a supplement, something to fall back on in times of emergency. The Lord didn't want his children to be tied to one kind of food, so that if it failed, mankind would die. Instead we are able to eat practically anything. But just because we *can* eat practically anything, doesn't mean that we're *meant* to eat practically everything.

One of the chief similarities between human systems and those of carnivores is the length of the colon. Carnivores tend to have large, short, and comparatively smooth bowels. However, in most grazing animals the bowel is long and convoluted. The reason is simply that if the meat stayed in the bowel of the carnivore for any great length of time, the putrefaction would kill it, while the grazing animals need longer to get the full value of the grasses and grains they eat — and there's no hurry to digest the grain before it kills them.

The human colon, at first glance, seems short, like that of the carnivore. "Aha!" say the meat advocates, "man was meant to eat meat!"

"Aha!" say those who look closer, "it just ain't true!"

The human colon is actually rather long, after all. However, it is foreshortened by three ribbonlike muscle bands running the length of the organ. The human colon can — and does — stretch. And it is therefore an ideal organ for digesting fruits, nuts, grains, and vegetables. On the other hand, food takes a long time passing through the human bowel. Long enough for meat to cause harm.

Furthermore, the human intestine has all the convolutions of the herbivore's bowel; and the closer you look, the more you realize that while humans are capable of eating practically anything, they were *meant* to eat vegetables.

If more comparisons are needed, man's dental structure again points to our intended vegetable diet. We lack the grasping, tearing teeth of true carnivores — take a good look at the teeth of your dog or your cat to see what a meat-eater's teeth look like. Instead, human beings have the sharp, flat, scissorlike incisors meant for biting off digestible pieces of fruits and vegetables. We have the flat, nodular molars that are best for grinding grains, nuts, and vegetables into pieces small enough to swallow.

Man is clearly designed to eat vegetables, points out W. S. Collens, but we have perverted our dietary habits with too, too much meat. "Herein may lie the basis for the high incidence of human atherosclerotic disease." (Collens and G. B. Dobkin, "Phylogenetic Aspects of the Cause of Human Atherosclerotic Disease," *Circulation*, Suppl. 2, 32:7, Oct. 1975.)

And when human beings eat meat, the stomach secretes much more of the peptic acid and other gastric juices than when vegetables are being digested. Those peptic acids, in high enough concentration, are the cause of stomach ulcers.

And just in case you're still in the mood to take all the kids out for a hamburger whenever you're in a hurry, remember a recent finding at the University of California, San Francisco. Pediatricians there have discovered that too much acidity in the body severely stunts the growth of young children. The children they were working with had a kidney disease that caused their violently excess acidity; the children were far undersize for their age. Because the disease was severe, they took stringent methods to reduce acidity — regular doses of baking soda.

The acidity of the human body rises as more meat is eaten. And while overuse of meat doesn't cause the severe stunting of growth that these children's kidney disease causes, it can still slow the early growth processes. And if the acidity isn't reversed while the children are still quite young, the loss of growth can't be made up.

The very young aren't the only ones who suffer from the consequences of "over-meating." People of middle age and beyond just don't have digestive systems to handle much meat. Proteins in large quantities build up nitrogen in the blood, which has to be discharged by the kidneys. But the kidneys, long overworked, just can't handle the load, and the nitrogen-containing waste builds up, causing high blood pressure, among other things.

Too much protein, too quickly ingested, can cause a negative calcium balance. (Too little protein, of course, causes the opposite problem — an inability to retain the calcium that is eaten.)

At the same time, meat is not utterly harmful — obviously not, since many meat-eaters live to a ripe old age. Meat does contain nutrients in large quantities; in times of cold, or when no other food is available, meat is certainly a viable alternative. But meat, in large quantities and over a long period of time, does have a debilitating effect on the human body.

When is meat most valuable to us? In cold weather, meat's putrefying qualities are less harmful, and therefore meat is safer to eat. And in famine, when the body needs protein to keep tissues alive, meat certainly does *that* job.

But eating meat in other times just gives us excess protein, which has to be eliminated from the body, causing strain. And the Lord was pretty clear when he said, "Wo be unto man that sheddeth blood or that wasteth flesh and hath no need." (D&C 49:21.) When you eat 40 percent more protein than your body needs, that protein is wasted. When every meal includes animal flesh, when ample nutrients are avail-

able from other, more healthful sources, someone had shed
blood who "hath no need."

The Word of Wisdom does not counsel vegetarianism.
Animals are on the earth for the use of man — when man
needs them. But when they aren't needed — which is most of
the time — the human diet should be based on grains, vegetables, and fruits, the diet of the Garden of Eden, and not on
the flesh of animals.

Meat animals "hath God made for the use of man only in
times of famine and excess of hunger." (D&C 89:15.) Heard of
any famines lately? And how long has it been since you were
excessively hungry?

5

What Sugar Does to You Isn't So Sweet

Sugar is a miracle food, they tell us. Sugar, refined and rerefined until it's 100 percent pure carbohydrate, pours more energy into our bloodstream than any other food. Why, it's practically predigested! All that energy — sounds wonderful, doesn't it?

Unless you stop and realize that if there was ever a time in history when large amounts of energy were *not* needed in our bloodstreams, it's now! Even if you exercise regularly, chances are pretty slim that you're using up so much energy so quickly that you can possibly utilize all the energy in the sugar in one cupcake!

What happened to that flood of sugar that came from that presweetened breakfast cereal or that candy bar or that pastry you just had for dessert?

Unless you immediately ran outside and did a few miles of running (which isn't the world's best idea right after eating!) that sugar coursed through your bloodstream uselessly, utterly unneeded by your body cells. Then, because it was there and had to be absorbed, it was taken into your body in the one place you didn't want it — in your fat cells.

And there it stays — because when your body needs energy again, it won't draw the stored energy out of your fat cells, it will draw it from the more slowly digested starches, which provide usable carbohydrates at a much slower rate. And all that wonderful instant energy from the sugar you ate turns into fat, which isn't very instant at all!

When Joseph Smith received the Word of Wisdom from the Lord, sugar wasn't generally known — at least not in the refined state it is in today. Since that time, sugar has become an increasingly important part of our regular diet — and it has, in the meantime, become so refined that none of the vitamins and minerals that were originally in the sugar beet or the sugar cane survive to come to our table.

Sugar is pure.

Which means that it has been refined into the most useless food imaginable — instant energy for a society that uses less energy than any other in the history of the world.

While much of the nutritional value of wheat is stripped away in refining it to white flour, it still contains many different nutrients, and does make a contribution to the diet, including complex carbohydrates (starches), protein, and those other nutrients restored in the "enriching process." Sugar, on the other hand, provides absolutely nothing but energy in its most accessible form. It contains nothing that can build the body at all — it can only be burned off or stored as fat. That is why, though white flour, used as the only source of wheat, can be debilitating, I still class it as a "fair food" — while sugar is downright bad. What is a good food? Why, one that still retains every natural benefit it can give to man.

It's hard to find a natural benefit from sugar.

And yet it might be possible to overlook sugar if uselessness were its only feature. Sugar, however, is harmful.

The evidence linking high sugar intake to diabetes is irrefutable. In 1971, Dr. D. G. Campbell published his conviction that, after long years of study, only one conclusion about sugar is reasonable: It can kill. And those who survive are seriously weakened by it.

What are some of his findings?

The onset of diabetes is commonest after twenty years of high sugar (sucrose) intake.

Tropical countries where diabetes is a common disease invariably have an annual per capita sugar intake of more than seventy pounds.

In any group of people whose caloric intake is low — less than 2,400 calories per day — yet where diabetes is common, the sucrose intake always exceeds 20 percent of the total caloric intake. (D. G. Campbell, *Addiction to Sugar,* Geigy Pharmaceuticals, Montreal, 1971.)

How much sugar do *we* eat?

Right now in America, sugar represents 16.4 percent of the caloric intake. But we eat more calories — and so our sugar intake in absolute numbers far outstrips the meager seventy pounds per person per year that Dr. Campbell found in diabetes-prone tropical countries.

We eat more than 100 pounds per person every year! That's about a quarter pound a day.

But wait a minute! *You* don't eat that much sugar, do you?

Sugar has a way of sneaking into many different foods. Sugar doesn't always come as white or brown powder that you sprinkle onto breakfast cereal. Sugar also comes in many other forms.

Jam on your toast is almost entirely sugar.

Canned fruit contains high concentrations of sugar.

Syrup on pancakes is almost pure sugar.

Soft drinks are almost entirely sugar.

Every cake, candy, donut, cooky, or "breath mint" you eat is mostly sugar, so far as the calories it provides are concerned.

And sugar creeps into hundreds of other foods, too.

Why is sugar so heavily used? The simple answer is that the public demands sugar. We have a sweet tooth — we want foods with sugar in them, and we pay to get them. It would be a foolish businessman who didn't recognize that fact and take advantage of it.

And why do we crave sugar so much? After all, our ancestors of only a few hundred years ago didn't know what sugar was, by and large, and rarely had sweets as we know them today.

We want so much sugar because we eat so much sugar. Sugar is its own reinforcer. When we eat sugar, it forces the pancreas to produce more insulin in order to digest it. Then the sugar enters the bloodstream, and then, very quickly, passes out again, absorbed by the body, sometimes as energy, but more often as fat deposits.

However, the pancreatic fluids don't pass out of the bloodstream that quickly. The overload of sugar causes an overload of pancreatic secretions — and these, remaining in the bloodstream long after the sugar has gone, signal the brain that more sugar is needed to use them up. An hour or so after eating a candy bar, we want another, because the massive dose of sugar we have just taken fools the body into thinking it has a sugar *deficiency*.

It's a vicious circle: large amounts of sugar force the body to produce large amounts of digestive fluid. The pancreatic secretions remain in the blood longer than the sugar. The presence of pancreatic secretions without a lot of sugar in the blood signals the body that sugar is needed. And we find ourselves heading for the candy machine, the cooky jar, or the jampot.

Of course, complex carbohydrates, often called starches, are the basis of some of the most valuable food we have — wheat, potatoes, legumes, and many others. Aren't they, too, dangerous? After all, the entire digestive process works to break these complex carbohydrates down into sugars — which enter the bloodstream just the way sucrose does.

In fact, overeating starches can cause just as much sugar overload as eating sugar, and the excess energy goes straight into fat. However, starches don't have the same negative effect that sugar has simply because they *are* complex molecules, and it takes the body longer to digest them. Where sugar enters the bloodstream quickly, overtaxing the pancreas and disrupting normal body functions, starches are digested more slowly, and enter the bloodstream gradually, not causing anywhere near the strain on the body's organs. Starches can contribute to overweight — but there is no evidence linking them to hypoglycemia (low blood sugar, a forerunner of diabetes in many cases) and diabetes, while with sugar there is no doubt about the close relationship between overuse and pancreatic malfunction.

Because sugar is self-reinforcing, its use builds up over a long period of time, and we can become virtually addicted to it. Many heavy sugar-eaters have reported that when going on a diet that required abstinence from sugar, they suffer severe headaches and light-headedness — problems that were instantly cured by eating sugar. If you are so dependent on sugar that cutting out sweets causes you withdrawal symptoms, just like those of any other addict, chances are pretty good that you've been eating far too much sugar — and it's time to quit!

Besides hypoglycemia and diabetes, overuse of sugar has been linked with other body conditions. Gas in the stomach and bowel is a common complaint in our society — obviously, or drug manufacturers would not spend so much time advertising cures for the complaint. Sugar is a leading cause of gassiness.

Sugar also had been linked with atherosclerosis, a condition long blamed on eggs and other high cholesterol foods. Several experiments have been performed, trying to find out what causes some people who eat normal amounts of cholesterol to have cholesterol build-ups in their arteries, while others, who eat more cholesterol, don't have a bloodstream highly charged with the substance. And one of the linchpins in atherosclerosis seems to be sugar.

When human subjects replaced sugar in their diet with more complex carbohydrates, there was a definite decrease in the concentration of cholesterol and glycerides in the bloodstream.

Subjects eating a diet largely built around sugar complained of frequent hunger, regardless of how much they ate — that vicious circle of self-reinforcement again. Those on the diet of starches, however, felt stuffed, and didn't crave so many between-meal snacks.

Another factor that seemed important was the balance of meals during the day. Those who ate three equal meals a day had lower (and therefore more healthy) cholesterol and glyceride concentrations in the blood than those who followed our normal pattern of three unequal meals. (Robert E. Hodges, M.D., and W. A. Krehl, M.D., "The Role of Carbohydrate in Lipid Metabolism," *American Journal of Clinical Nutrition*, Nov. 1965, 17:334-46.)

And while researchers disagree acutely on the question of whether high sugar intake is related to heart disease, enough evidence exists to convince many researchers, and to lead even those who doubt that link to say things like this: "There are plenty of good arguments to reduce the flood of dietary sucrose without building a mountain of nonsense about coronary heart disease." (Ancel Keys, "Sucrose in the Diet and Coronary Heart Disease," *Atherosclerosis*, Amsterdam: Elsevier.)

The complex patterns of metabolism — the body's burning of energy taken in as food — are not yet fully understood, but Bender and Thadani in studies published in 1970 found that sucrose — commercial sugar — depressed the rate at which the body was able to burn up glucose, the sugar that results from the digestion of starches. In other words, the sugar you eat makes it harder for your body to use the much more valuable carbohydrates in grains, legumes, and other vegetables. (A. E. Bender and Pushpa V. Thadani, "Some Metabolic Effects of Dietary Sucrose," *Nutrition and Metabolism*, 1970, 12:22-39.)

Dr. Lauren V. Ackerman, a prize-winning researcher in causes of cancer, has begun to suspect sugar and other highly refined foods in Western man's diet as a leading cause of cancer. After all, cancer is nowhere near as prevalent among more "primitive" societies that stay away from refined foods. Dr. Ackerman has said: "It does not seem too much to assert that 80 percent of all cancers are related to one or more factors in man's environment." And one of the main factors is our overdependence on refined foods. "The replacement of un-refined carbohydrates, such as cereals, corn products, and brown [whole wheat] bread, by refined carbohydrates, such as sugar and white flour, in our diet may well be responsible for the steadily increasing incidence of cancer of the large bowel we see in North America. . . .

"In my opinion, it has been demonstrated beyond any doubt that the environmental factor of nutrition contributes in significant measure to the genesis of the second most lethal cancer in North American, cancer of the large intestine." (Ackerman, "Some Thoughts on Food and Cancer," *Nutrition Today,* Jan./Dec. 1972.)

The most lethal cancer in America is cancer of the lung, largely self-inflicted because of pathological dependence on tobacco. Latter-day Saints are largely free of that disease. However, we save our lives only to run the risk of cancer of the intestine — because of a pathological dependence on sugar and other refined foods!

It is no accident, either, that the American Heart Association recommends four changes in our diet to avoid heart disease — and one of those changes is to substitute natural starch for sugar as our source of carbohydrate. If this recommendation were taken it would automatically help cure obesity, since we wouldn't have the constant hunger that sugar induces; and curing obesity is one of the best ways to avoid heart trouble.

There are those who, unfortunately, believe that if anything overrefined is bad for you, then anything that is not refined must be good for you. While this is true in some cases, it is definitely *not* true in the case of sugar. Brown sugar is no less dangerous than white sugar — nor is "raw" sugar. They all provide instant sucrose for the body and have precisely the same effects on the bloodstream and the pancreas. They are no more "natural" and beneficial in our diet than pure refined white sugar. Even though brown sugar and raw sugar have traces of other nutrients that white sugar lacks, practically any other food in the world provides more of those nutrients than raw sugar provides — while raw sugar still has all the harmful effects of white sugar.

Even honey, often touted as a good sugar substitute, is a quick energy source which, if used heavily, would have precisely the same effect on the body as white sugar. The only reason that brown and raw sugar and honey aren't so roundly condemned as white sugar is that we don't eat as much of them as we do of white sugar. But if we were to replace all our white sugar intake with brown sugar and honey, and ate them in as great a quantity as we do white sugar, we wouldn't have helped our health at all.

The only cure for our overdependence on sugar is simply to cut down drastically on how much of it we eat. That wouldn't mean utterly eliminating sugars from our diet. But the sweetness found in nutrient-rich fruits should be more than enough for us, since their sugar content is certainly high enough to satisfy any reasonable desire for sweets, while they have enough nutrients to make them a valuable food.

Giving up sugar sounds hard to many people — and yet to many skeptics it sounds far too easy." You mean that cutting out sugar will help cure diabetes, cancer, and heart disease? That sounds like a patent medicine, not a serious scientific finding," the skeptics say. But besides helping cut down on the chances of tooth decay, eliminating sugar, as much as possible, from the diet really does increase your general health and resistance to the point where many diseases simply have no hold of you, while others are far less likely to occur.

All the effects of sugar are not known. But we do know that many, many people have eliminated it largely from their diet — and have discovered that sugar, the "miracle food," the source of "pure instant energy," had actually been dragging down their health for years; and without it, they got what patent medicines only promise — a new lease on life.

Who needs instant energy? The human body needs slow, carefully regulated, gradually usable energy. Instant energy in the form of sugar is like 220 volts applied to an appliance meant to run on 110 volts — destruction, not more power at all.

You don't need sugar, and it can hurt you. Doesn't make much sense, then, does it, to eat that candy bar? Or that cake? Here's a word of wisdom — when you want something sweet, eat a fruit. And after a while, the craving for sugar, like the dependence for any other addictive and harmful chemical, will go away and let you return to good health.

6

Fat People Are
Starving in America

"Eat all the food on your plate," insisted mothers who had known the hunger and insecurity of poverty during the Depression. "Eat every scrap. Children are starving in Europe."

And so a generation, and then another, grew up believing that if the food was *there* it should be eaten. And Americans grew fatter, and fatter, and fatter — because no matter how much they ate, there was always more food.

Yet despite the prevalence of obesity in America — conservative estimates place it as a problem with more than a fifth of the adult population — the very people who seem to be most overfed are starving.

Not for calories — they have calories to spare for some time to come.

They are starving for nutrients.

But aren't calories nutrients? No — not at all. Calories are a measurement for energy, and with food, they are usually counted as the potential energy in a certain amount of food, once it is digested and used by the body. But the body needs many things besides energy.

Though it takes energy to build a cell, it also takes the large building blocks or proteins and the smaller building blocks of trace elements like nitrogen, calcium, phosphorus, iron, and many others. Also, the body depends on incredibly complex enzymes and hormones to regulate life.

Energy in the body is like gasoline in a car. You can pour as much gasoline in the car as you like, but if the tires, the engine block, the battery, the starter, and all the other moving parts are in poor condition, that gasoline might as well be water. The car needs more than fuel to run properly.

Your body is much more complex than a car. And while we pump fuel into our bodies until it is, quite literally, poking out all over, we simultaneously neglect all the other aspects of maintaining our bodies in good working order.

We are overfed and undernourished.

In fact, undernourishment is one of the main causes of obesity. Our body has a delicate mechanism for telling us when we should eat. But we often don't know how to read that mechanism. When we are short on several vital chemicals needed to keep our body working, that mechanism triggers a feeling we recognize as hunger. But instead of providing the kind of food that will meet the body's needs, we often just pump in more poor-grade fuel: sugar, refined flour, shortening, and little else. The body doesn't feel satisfied for long — those chemicals are still urgently needed. And so while the huge amounts of energy that have been dumped into the body are converted resolutely into fat, the body again signals *hunger*.

And the person who just ate wonders why he can never seem to get enough food — and yet is gaining weight.

That is not, of course, the only reason why people gain weight. Some people have glandular conditions that force their bodies to convert more and more of the food they eat into fat. Other people simply have more fat cells than others — heredity did them no favor in our slim-worshipping society.

Still more people, however, eat because they're nervous, or because they're bored, or because they're afraid and insecure. They eat because they need to be doing *something* that makes them feel good. And chewing and swallowing, particularly if the food is sweet or spicy, makes them feel better. For a while. Of course, as the mirror shows more and more fat on their bodies, they feel even more insecure, even more nervous, and so to feel good they eat again. Another vicious circle, this time emotional.

There are two types of obesity. The first and most common is called *hypertrophy*. Hypertrophy is the abnormal growth of individual fat cells. Each cell becomes overloaded with fatty acids, the basic energy-storing chemical deposited as fat. And as all the individual fat cells grow, the body appears to be growing larger.

The second kind of obesity is *hyperplasia*. This is a very different condition, in which fat cells don't merely grow — they multiply, so that there are *more* fat cells rather than just larger fat cells.

Hyperplasia is not very well understood. It seems to be caused more by heredity, though recent findings indicate that overfed babies tend to lay down more fat cells in their formative years, and those fat cells are incredibly hard to get rid of.

The most common form of obesity, however, is hypertrophy, and it is also much easier to overcome. The cells that grew to distended proportions can be shrunk back to normal, performing the necessary function that fat performs in the body. (A body utterly without fat is commonly referred to as *starving*, and is usually close to death. What we call "fat" is usually simply too much fat.)

Overeating, however, is a relative thing. The body regularly raids fat cells for energy to use during activities. That is, after all, what fat cells are for — a system of tiny storage batteries to provide energy for the body on a regular basis. If a person uses a lot of energy because he leads an active life, the fuel put into fat cells as fatty acids will flow out as much as it flows in, and the person will not be obese.

However, a person who is not active, if he eats as much as an active person, will simply keep charging and recharging and charging again batteries in his body that he never uses.

There isn't a regular flow of energy into and out of fat cells — energy only flows in. And obesity is the inevitable result.

Does this mean that if you exercise drastically, you'll lose weight? It isn't quite that simple. Actually, if you start exercising you'll simply get hungrier, and your body will make more efficient use of the food you eat — but the pounds won't flow off. Exercise maintains your weight and keeps you in good shape — but once the weight is on, you have to change eating habits, besides exercising, in order to get a healthy fat balance in your body.

"I've lost three thousand pounds," many a dieter can claim. "Unfortunately, I've also gained three thousand fifty pounds."

Overweight people tend to fly back and forth between extremes. They try every diet they can — liquid protein, no carbohydrates, fasting, calorie counting, grapefruit and eggs, watermelon, glucose, gluten — anything. And practically every diet works. The pounds come off fast — far too fast for the body's good. And then, as the formerly obese person reaches the desired weight, he or she breathes a sigh of relief, buys a new wardrobe, and then has four ice cream cones, two pies, and thirty-seven candy bars to celebrate.

The weight goes on again just as quickly as it came off.

Actually, it's more harmful on the body to have rapid weight fluctuations of any large amount than it is to be obese! For a diet to do any good, it needs to take the weight off and keep it off. A fat person can't regard a diet as a phase he must pass through, only to return to the coveted habits of overeating. A good diet is simply sensible eating — a lifetime habit of carefully eating only as much as is necessary, and no more.

When you're taking off weight, you're playing with your body's starvation mechanisms. For instance, if you go on a crash diet that only allows you one meal a day, your body regards that as deprivation, and immediately begins to compensate — by storing up every calorie that comes in as fat. The diet actually encourages your body to hang onto every ounce of fat it can.

Instead, a good weight-loss diet provides three small

meals a day. Those meals need to be nutritionally balanced. Liquid protein is known to kill, and other diets that restrict their victims to strange combinations of food — or only one type of food at all — actually do induce a condition of starvation in the body. Starvation sets off every alarm that the body has. It's an emergency condition, and the body starts to function poorly. Ill health is the inevitable result. And when the diet is over, the body immediately demands a return of equilibrium, which usually means all the bad habits from before.

A balanced diet, however, will give the body all the nutrients it needs — all the vitamins and minerals necessary for normal body functions to take place. The only difference between a weight-loss diet and a normal healthy diet is that the weight-loss diet will not provide enough *calories* for the body's normal needs, while it still provides everything else the body must have. After all, the only thing that makes you fat is the accumulation of fatty acids, and a chemical reaction can be induced to cause these fatty acids to be released as energy. By giving your body less energy than it needs, while providing everything else, the molecules of fatty acids break down to make up the deficiency. Your body doesn't go into overdrive because it thinks it's being starved to death. And the pounds go off, not dramatically, but slowly and, most important, permanently.

Naturally, an increase in body activity will increase the amount of energy your body uses up. And if you're still eating balanced, nutritious meals, however small they might be, your body will feel up to carrying on those activities, taking energy from your fat supply all the time.

However, exercise is only a help, and it's more important in improving health and muscle tone than it is in weight loss. Why? Because unless you're a professional athlete working out for hours a day, you can't use up enough energy to make that much difference. Just staying alive takes between two and three thousand calories a day. Normal exercise only increases that by about three or four hundred calories. An athlete might go so far as to double that requirement. But the basic caloric requirement must be regularly met, regardless of exercise, and that is the requirement that you must deal with in losing weight.

A pound of fat represents 3,500 calories. You have to jog a lot of miles to use up that much energy — but if you simply cut down five hundred calories a day, by the end of a week you'll have lost a pound. That isn't a terribly exciting weight loss — until you realize that cutting down five hundred calories a day is really quite painless. You can probably do it by making a dietary change you should have made long ago, like eliminating sugar from your diet! In fact, you can cut out five hundred calories by eating well-balanced meals of a size that should be ample for your eating pattern for the rest of your life.

And a pound a week is more than enough, as long as the weight stays off. In a year you can have lost as much as fifty-two pounds at that rate, though chances are good that you'll level off several times during the weight-loss process. And when you reach the weight that's healthy for your build and height, you can gradually increase your calories until you have just enough to maintain that weight, with a healthy amount of exercise.

The only diet that works, to put it simply, is a diet that changes your life. It is your lifestyle that put the pounds on you; only a change in that lifestyle can take them off.

Of course, on such a program the weight loss is so gradual that as you step on the scales you may feel that nothing is happening at all. Your body can fluctuate more than a pound in a single day, simply because of the amount of water being retained or given off. And so from one day to the next, it may seem that no progress is being made. That's why fad diets are so popular — they give quick, easily seen results. They also wreck your body, but that doesn't show up on the scale. When you're on a sensible diet, though, the scale will only tell part of the story, and then only over an extended period of time. The rest of the story will come as you find yourself feeling less hungry (those well-balanced meals again!), more healthy and vigorous, more energetic, and less weary and irritable. And you'll find yourself fitting back into the wardrobe that you haven't been able to button up in years.

It takes patience. It takes a serious commitment to good

health. And it pays off in health, better personal appearance, and an assurance that you're taking good care of the magnificent tabernacle your Father gave you for your second estate.

Parents should also take special care to make sure that patterns of obesity aren't established in their children. Children are much more responsive to their bodies' needs than adults usually are. If they don't need any more food, they simply stop eating — unless they're forced to continue. Parents' concern shouldn't be the *amount* that children eat, but rather *what* they eat. If children are given good, well-balanced meals, a minimum of sweets, and as much whole, unrefined grain as possible instead of overrefined foods, they will learn to enjoy those foods, and when their body tells them they aren't hungry anymore and they stop eating, parents can be confident that the child is well nourished.

One of the worst things that can be done to a child is to teach him that sweets are somehow linked with good behavior. If children are "rewarded" with ice cream, candy, or cake, or if sugary or overrefined foods like cakes, candies, jams, syrups, honey, and ice cream are always linked with special occasions and fun times, children will come to think of those foods as especially fun or desirable. They should be taught to think of them as social necessities to avoid offending other people when visiting with them — but in their own home, children should learn to relish wholesome foods as their treats or rewards — if rewards have to be linked to eating at all!

The child who is raised believing that the best thing that can happen at a family party is for a plate of apples and pears to be passed around is a child who is far less likely to be overweight as an adult than the poor child who has to have a slice of cake a la mode before he feels that the party is complete. Unfortunately, most parents are themselves the victims of seemingly insatiable cravings for sweets. It's hard for them to be very convincing when they tell their children how wonderful their celery and brussels sprouts are, because they crave a candy bar just as much as their children do!

Contrary to popular myth, many children have actually grown to adulthood without trauma or terrible emotional problems — *without* having learned to love sweets.

But they can't very well do it in a home where parents eat foolishly. So you owe it, not only to yourselves, but also to your children to have a regular healthy diet of the right kinds of foods. Your weight problems will be over — and your children will never have them at all.

7

What You Don't Eat Can Make You Sick

"Supernutrition," Dr. Roger J. Williams called it, and he said it may prevent cancer and other diseases. Supernutrition goes beyond merely counting calories, beyond merely sensible nutrition. "It deserves investigation as a strategy for the control of disease."

Dr. Williams was not a health food quack preaching a panacea to a group of gullible onlookers. Instead he was delivering a scientific paper to the National Academy of Sciences. And what he was talking about was not a single "health" food, but rather a complex series of disease prevention techniques through the use of nutrition.

Why had Williams come to view nutrition — or supernutrition — as the key to disease prevention? The experiments forced him to that conclusion:

Two-thirds of a group of rats fed only on commercial white bread died within ninety days — of malnutrition. The few survivors were severely stunted. Yet the same rats could have survived quite well for a long time on a diet of uncooked wheat. In his report to the academy, Williams declared that he suspected there were unknown but significant nutrients or combinations of nutrients in unrefined, uncooked foods — nutrients that may be desperately needed by human beings.

He described another experiment: "A group of mice already receiving a commercial stock diet, supposedly well supplied with all nutrients, including pantothenic acid, were given an extra supply of calcium pantothenate in their drinking water. The result was an increased longevity of about 19 percent. If this result is achieved by strengthening only one link in the chain, one can legitimately expect the result to be even more striking if one attempted to strengthen all the links."

That was why Williams was willing to publicly state that he suspected a link between supernutrition — increasing doses of key nutrients — to be a key to the prevention of such diseases as muscular dystrophy, multiple sclerosis, and cancer. And the effects would, logically, be more pronounced if supernutrition were begun at a very early age.

"There is certainly room for the hypothesis that cells will not go [become cancerous] if they are continuously supported by strong environmental conditions," said Williams. But so far no one has tried using supernutrition on human beings — partly because it would take literally five or six decades before the results of supernutrition begun at an early age could be measured in terms of fewer cases of cancer in late adulthood. Once again, the short lifespan of rats makes them much better research subjects than human beings.

Williams isn't talking, of course, about some magical food or substance that will mysteriously bring a person to the peak of health. Rather, he's suggesting that simply increasing the amounts of key nutrients already well known as necessary to the body, while emphasizing whole, uncooked foods in the diet, may prevent diseases that seem now to be unstoppable.

The "cures" for cancer and other diseases, when there's a cure at all, are usually drastic and devastating — removal of organs, radiation treatments, and so on. Wouldn't it be better to stop those diseases from beginning at all? Prevention is the best cure; but the business of physicians is treatment, not prevention. Your doctor doesn't get called until there's a problem. But if you, by changing the way you eat, could keep yourself so healthy you never needed the doctor at all, you'd be far, far better off.

Of course, we don't know enough about nutrition yet. The experiments haven't been performed, the results aren't in. But by the time all the findings are established and published, you'll probably be dead! So why not live by the best knowledge available today in caring for the body the Lord has entrusted to you?

Supernutrition is still in your future — but right now you can at least be following good principles of that rare thing called "normal" nutrition in your daily diet.

If you desire the best health available according to our best knowledge today, these are the principles you should be following in your diet:

1. Abstain from all the items specifically forbidden in the Word of Wisdom: alcohol, tea, coffee, and tobacco. By extension, it would be wise to generalize from those prohibitions and refrain from taking into your body *every* popular drug that upsets your body's metabolism and makes changes — as yet unmeasured — in your health. It would be good to avoid soft drinks containing caffeine, chocolate — which contains substances besides caffeine which can be harmful — harmful drugs of all kinds, and even self-prescribed medicines. The more rarely you use drugstore medicines, the more likely they'll be to help you when you *really* need them — and the less likely they are to do you unmeasured harm.

2. Drink freely of pure, fresh water. Plenty of water between meals reduces your desire for large amounts with meals.

3. Eat all wholesome foods regularly. Fruits, vegetables, legumes, occasionally nuts, balanced with whole grains, unrefined cereals, and other whole-grain products can be eaten, the Lord says, "with thanksgiving." They will assure you of an ample supply of energy, maintenance, and growth-promoting nutrients, along with vitamins and minerals accompanied by the complex systems the Lord created for our benefit.

4. Choose a variety of foods. As soon as you limit your diet

to two or three kinds of food, you are cutting down your chances of getting everything your body needs. Nutrition, despite recent advances, is still in many cases a guessing game. You can cover all the bases simply by making sure you don't cut yourself off from any of the herbs and fruits the Lord intended us to eat.

5. However, don't try to get all the variety in one meal! If you have eighteen different kinds of food on the table, all of them good, you'll probably eat some of everything — and that inevitably leads to overeating.

6. Avoid refined foods wherever possible. Even when they purport to be enriched with vitamins and minerals, the refining and enriching process replaces vitamins and minerals in a natural setting, with all the accompanying enzymes and nutrient complexes, with sterile, refined vitamins and minerals that simply don't act in your body the way they should. And refined foods are hard on your digestion.

7. Sugar should be regarded as potentially dangerous. If you want something sweet, eat fruit that contains natural sugar in a good proportion to other nutrients. When you sprinkle sugar — white or brown — on any food, or when you mix it into a batter, or when you spread a sugar product on bread, you are giving your body a jolt of pure energy. If you wouldn't stick your finger into a light socket, don't dump extra, potentially harmful energy into your body!

8. Regard meat as a supplemental food, to be eaten only when you need it. And you don't need it very often! Meat can cause you harm, especially when you eat it regularly. You can have a completely balanced diet without it. And if you feel that you do need some meat products, stick to milk and eggs before you turn to muscle meat.

9. Eat meals regularly, and make sure that you're rested and relaxed during your meals. Meals eaten in a hurry or under emotional stress are affected by the chemicals that your body releases when you're tense. Don't ruin the chances of a good meal by being in turmoil while you eat it!

10. Balance your meals throughout the day. Breakfast, lunch, and dinner should each supply about a third of your

daily nutrients. And if you want to skimp on any meal, take a light supper, giving the digestive system a chance to rest during the night.

11. Don't eat much between meals. This is especially true for adults, who aren't, we hope, growing. You just don't need those extra calories. If you start getting a little hungry between meals, it's a good sign — it means you're getting off the habit of constantly gorging yourself, and your body is noticing. After a while of eating regularly and carefully, your body will only signal you that it's hungry when you really *should* eat.

12. No matter how healthful a food might be, eating too much of it only overloads your system and causes you to build up fat, which can create a terrible strain on the body. It's not just the heart that suffers from overeating — your liver and kidneys are also forced into overtime work when you eat more than you need. It's a good idea to leave the table while the food still looks good to you, instead of staggering away bloated, wondering if you can make it to the living room couch to lie down and recover from your marathon meal. Besides, when you eat too much your stomach is too full to work properly. Digestion slows down, and fermentation is more likely, leading to all kinds of potential diseases.

The average person eats:

Too much!

Too much meat.

Too many sweets.

Too many refined foods.

Too little whole food — grains and cereals, the staff of life.

Too few fresh fruits and vegetables.

Remember that every serving of junk food you eat crowds out a serving you might have had of heathful, balanced food.

And then, once you've gotten in the habit of eating properly, your body will be much more ready to take the other step in obeying the Word of Wisdom and caring for the body the Lord gave you: exercise.

II

Exercising Intelligently

Physical fitness is more than a passing fad or an occasional activity. Physical fitness means keeping your body constantly in good enough shape to perform your normal daily work and play – and still have a reserve to meet unexpected demands on your strength, your physical skills, and your endurance. If you haven't been keeping your body in use, it won't be usable when you desperately need it.

8

Who Has Time to Exercise?

Suppose you live 25,000 days. That's nearly seventy years, certainly a normal life expectancy. In those days, you'll have 613,200 hours. If you knew that by spending only 4 percent of that time in vigorous exercise, you could make the other 96 percent of those hours more healthful, more pleasant, and more productive — and probably add another 90,000 hours to your life — wouldn't you regard that as a good investment?

Over your lifetime, if you exercise vigorously for only an hour a day, that would add up to 25,000 hours in a normal lifespan. That exercise can add another ten or more vigorous years to your life — 90,000 more hours. That's almost a 300 percent return on your investment — good business in anyone's book.

But there are more dividends to exercise than just adding to your lifespan. Those who live a sedentary life, sitting most of the day and rarely getting more exercise than walking to the car and back or pushing a cart through a supermarket, usually find themselves by their mid-twenties feeling lethargic, lacking energy, not wishing to exercise any more than necessary.

They don't feel that way because they're tired — they feel that way because their bodies are slogging down into unfitness. They don't feel like vigorous exercise because they're no longer capable of vigorous exercise at a moment's notice.

By their mid-thirties, such people are already suffering from poor health because of lack of exercise. Constant sitting causes hard fat to deposit in unpleasant places. Muscles cramp easily, and aches and pains come rather frequently. Posture is poor, strength is virtually gone, and climbing stairs or running to catch a bus leaves such people panting, out of breath, exhausted. The muscle tone that makes a body attractive and beautiful is gone, and instead the body pouches, droops, sags — even if it isn't overweight.

By the mid-forties, the process is virtually complete, and diseases start to come. The strength and resistance to overcome them just isn't there anymore. Worse, during a person's most productive years; during the time when the children most need their parents to be vigorous; that is the very time when years of sedentary life have sapped the adult of his strength. His mind doesn't function very clearly anymore. He has a hard time concentrating. His emotions tend to be more negative, and he feels out of sorts all the time. Getting up in the morning is misery.

Life just isn't any fun.

All of this, because he couldn't spare 4 percent of his life to make the other 96 percent worth living!

Does exercise — or the lack of it — make that much difference in a person's life?

You bet it does!

The human body was designed to move. It would be a poor designer who built a machine with unnecessary moving parts. There isn't a joint in your body that you don't move — and often — from your jaws to your toes. All day you shake your head, move your jaw, lift your arms, crook your elbows, manipulate your wrists and fingers, sit down and stand up, bend your legs as you walk, and keep your balance by moving your ankles and toes.

You do all this in the course of even the most sedentary life. But the problem is, your body is designed so that the more you use those joints and the muscles that make them open and close, the easier it is to move them.

Muscles die from nonuse. If you lived for five years in bed, never lifting your arms or legs, never rolling over, never even opening your mouth to talk, then presuming you were still alive and still sane, you would discover that you hadn't the strength to lift yourself out of bed. You wouldn't be able to walk. You wouldn't be able to lift a glass of water to your mouth.

Even trying to move would be agony.

Unused muscles atrophy; cells die, and the muscles shrink. Our ancestors probably didn't know that — for thousands of years, men worked by using their muscles. Even those whose trade was sedentary had to walk or run long distances just to get from one place to another; even those wealthy enough to afford other means of transportation considered it a point of pride to be good horsemen, and riding a horse isn't a passive occupation.

Our ancestors didn't have to worry very much about muscle atrophy because they constantly used their muscles.

In our pushbutton instant age, however, it's possible to spend a whole week without having walked more than a hundred feet at a time. It's possible to go for years without lifting anything heavier than a grocery bag — and if it gets heavy enough, they carry it out to the car for you! It's possible to go for years without spending much time outdoors at all, as we go from air-conditioned house to air-conditioned car to air-conditioned office, stopping at air-conditioned stores on the way.

How long has it been since you've worked yourself into a good sweat? Since you've run so hard or played so vigorously that your muscles ached deliciously? Since you've had the strength to lift something heavier than a twenty-pound sack of flour? Since you've had the endurance to keep up a physical activity for more than a half hour?

But then, do we really *need* those muscles? We *do* live in a pushbutton age, after all — who *needs* to be as strong as our peasant ancestors?

In the terrible blizzards of 1977 and 1978, dozens of people lost their lives because they hadn't the strength to walk to safety in the cold and snow. Their strength gave out only a short way from their cars.

Imagine — if you were on a speedboat that collided with another in the middle of a lake, a mile from any shore, could you swim to safety?

If you were in an airplane that ditched in the ocean, would you have the stamina to stay afloat until rescuers came?

If your child were about to topple into a river or a ditch only fifty yards away, could you run fast enough to get there in time to save him from drowning?

If you had to pull your family out of a burning car, or carry unconscious family members out of your burning house, would you have the strength to lift them and move them quickly to safety?

Emergencies happen to people all the time — and an ever-decreasing number are in good enough physical shape to cope with them.

But even if you passed your life without a single emergency, muscle atrophy would be a serious problem because your heart is a muscle, and it atrophies along with everything else. Weak muscles can't help with the blood circulation, and you can become gouty or rheumatic; your veins can become varicose; you can be crippled.

All because you couldn't spare 4 percent of your time for exercise. Even 2 percent would be a great help. But you're just too busy to bother saving your own life, your own health, your own ability to enjoy your time on earth.

It wasn't all that long ago that our forefathers worked so long and so hard that they viewed physical labor as a necessity to be avoided whenever possible. They could afford to have that attitude, because it was rarely possible to avoid it!

We, on the other hand, should look at physical labor as a privilege to be seized upon whenever we can. If we take every opportunity for physical labor, our bodies, marvelous machines that they are, will take that exercise and turn it into more health, more strength.

We can't afford to be as lazy as our ancestors wished they could be. They needed rest. We need exercise.

9

The Saw That Sharpens Itself the More You Cut

The tools that man makes wear out. The more they're used, the more poorly they function. If they're well cared for, they can last a long time — but eventually, despite the best of care, they wear out.

However, the Lord builds better than man. Though life is meant to have an end, up to a certain point our bodies actually *improve* with use, as long as we nourish them properly. And the more we use our bodies, the better they respond to the demands we put on them.

Not everyone needs the same amount of exercise, of course. Everyone has a biological need for physical activity, but some need more than others. Few people, however, need less than a minimum of half an hour's vigorous exercise a day, and most people are better off with a full hour.

Just as important as intensity is consistency. If your body is not in good shape right now, exercising violently will put a strain on it. That strain is good — if it is followed by exercise the next day, and the next, and the next. As your body becomes used to the regular demands, it responds by increasing the number and strength of muscle cells in your body.

However, if you only exercise sporadically, you only get an occasional strain. Your body doesn't build up muscles — it only gets worn down, since the demands only come rarely and suddenly, and your body has no chance to adjust and build up.

Exercise hard and regularly — and over a long period of time. You were born in pretty good general health; as a child, you probably ran around and played so hard that you stayed in good shape. If you aren't in shape now, it's most likely a condition that has built up over the years since you entered adulthood. Whether you're overweight or merely flabby, it took you *time* to wear down your self-sharpening body, and it takes time to build it back up.

But one of the best things about the human body is that it's rarely too late to begin an exercise program. Though some people have irreversible diseases and others are so old that really strenuous exercise is out of the question, most people can, within a reasonably short time — three to four months — get their body back into good condition. After several years, their bodies can be in perfect shape, despite the years of abuse and neglect that they went through before.

Your body is very forgiving. As soon as you repent of mistreating it, your body will start treating *you* better — and it gets even better every day.

What does exercise actually do to your body?

One of the first things that exercise affects is your heart. Muscles that are being actively used require oxygen and other nutrients. They get those nutrients from the blood, and as more nutrients are required during exercise, more blood has to pass through the arteries and veins leading to and coming from the muscles. Since the number of blood vessels can't immediately increase, the blood must pulse through the existing vessels faster — and that means the heart rate goes up.

When you begin an exercise program after a long period of neglect, your heart is as atrophied as the rest of your body. The heart rate zooms to a high level, and it takes a long time after you quit exercising for your heart to settle down to preexercise levels. However, when you exercise regularly over a long period of time, and vigorously enough that your heart is forced to work hard, a surprising thing happens. To get the same amount of blood to your muscles, your heart doesn't have to beat as fast. Why not? Because the heart, which is a strong muscle to begin with, has become even stronger, each beat of the heart is able to carry more blood and push it harder through the vessels. Thus the heart doesn't have to beat weakly many times a minute — it can accomplish the same task now by beating more slowly, but with more force.

In other words, when you vigorously exercise the muscles of your body, your heart gets exercise, too, and soon it grows stronger and gets in better shape just as your other muscles do. Not only that, its endurance is better.

As the amount of blood pumped per heartbeat, or *stroke volume*, increases, the system of veins and arteries that make up the circulatory system also improves. As muscles develop, new blood vessels are gradually created to carry blood to and from them. As stroke volume increases, the blood vessels become stronger, able to bear greater amounts of blood.

Also, exercise improves the quality of blood. Because more oxygen is needed, the number of red blood cells increases, and makes up a higher proportion of any given amount of blood. There is more blood circulating. And the hemoglobin in the red blood cells, the substance that carries the oxygen, increases, too.

At what point does exercise have these beneficial effects on the heart and circulatory system? If you take a slow walk for exercise, it may develop your muscles, but it won't bring your heart to a level where it starts to improve. The level of exertion where the heart begins to develop is called the "critical threshold value," and in most people that comes when the heart rate is 60 percent of the way between the resting rate and the rate of maximum exertion. For instance, if your resting heart rate is 70 beats per minute, and your maximum heart rate when you're really exerting yourself is 200 beats per minute, then you subtract your resting rate from your maximum rate, which gives you 130 beats per minute, and find out what 60 percent of that is — 78 beats per minute. Add that figure to your resting heart rate, which gives you 148 beats per minute, and you have your critical threshold value. From then on, whenever you exercise vigorously enough that your heartbeat rate goes over 148 beats per minute for more than ten minutes, you are actually improving the performance of your heart. (If you have a preexisting heart problem, however, get your doctor's advice before starting an exercise program.)

How can you check your heartbeat? You don't have to count all the beats in a minute. Just find your pulse (in your wrist or your throat) and count how many beats there are in ten seconds. Then multiply by six. If you count eleven beats in ten seconds, that means your heartbeat rate is sixty-six beats per minute. (Some prefer to count the beats for fifteen seconds and multiply by four.)

When you regularly exercise at levels above your critical threshold value (called *aerobic exercise*) amazing things happen to your heart. First, the blood vessels that feed your heart increase in number and size, just like the blood vessels to any muscle that's getting lots of exercise. Having more coronary arteries means a much lower chance of heart attacks — and a much higher chance of recovery if you *should* have one.

Second, the tiny muscles that line all the veins and arteries in your body become stronger, because they, too, are getting exercise. They are exercised both because of the rhythmic contractions of the skeletal muscles through which they pass, and because of the stretching and tension caused by blood moving faster through the vessels.

Third, as your heart and blood vessels increase their capacity, high blood pressure gradually decreases toward normal. And any excess cholesterol and lipids in your bloodstream are dissipated, decreasing your chances of atherosclerosis.

Exercise has good effects on other systems, too. The lungs are one of the key points in physical fitness. The amount of oxygen that can be transferred from the air to the bloodstream across the thin barrier of the tiny alveoli in the lungs is the barrier that limits how much physical work we can do. When the oxygen runs out or runs low, the work stops or slows down.

Exercise helps increase the lungs' capacity in two ways. First, it strengthens the muscles involved in drawing in and expelling air, which allows ever greater amounts of air to be processed. Second, exercise improves the efficiency with which the air we do inhale is used by the lungs. Exercise is especially helpful if we are conscious of breathing deeply, forcing air ever deeper into the lungs, and bringing into action alveoli that have long had nothing to do — because air never got to them.

The digestive system is one body system that is not greatly affected by exercise — unless you make the mistake of engaging in strenuous exercise right after eating. The digestive system takes energy to function, partly because much of the work is done by muscles as food is churned in the stomach and passed by peristalsis through the intestines, and partly because the body has to produce digestive chemicals and enzymes to process the food. Also, as food is digested, it is passed into the blood, and while you are digesting food, your digestive system requires a large amount of blood.

That means that if you put a strain on your body during the initial stages of digestion, you are robbing the digestive system of some of the blood and oxygen it needs. The result can be severe stomach cramps — and failing that, your food will certainly not be digested properly.

However, if you exercise at other times, no harm will be done to your digestion, and the generally increased fitness of your body will obviously increase the digestive system's ability to function well.

When you exercise vigorously, you sweat. That's your body's way of passing off excess heat — through the evaporation of water on your body's surface. Also, sweating does have a cleansing effect, as salts and water are passed out of your system. The more you perspire, the more efficiently the perspiration system works.

In fact, your entire body works by the overload system. When organs and tissues are taxed beyond their capacity, the body's complex balancing systems force those organs and tissues to increase their capacity to meet the demand. Some organs, of course, are exceptions to the rule — there is no evidence that the brain, liver, or kidneys improve with over-load. However, exercise of the body's muscles doesn't over-load these three vital organs. In fact, because of the improve-ment in the heart and circulatory system, they function better because of physical exercise. The only way we can harmfully overload our kidneys or liver is by eating improperly — and since no one has yet fathomed the limits of the brain, there is no evidence that it's possible to overwork the brain itself, except through lack of sleep.

Have you ever had trouble getting to sleep? It's a rare person who exercises thoroughly who has any trouble getting to sleep. It's only when the brain is exhausted but the body isn't tired that you find yourself having problems sleeping as much as you need. The story is probably apocryphal, but has a foundation of truth: A lady complained to her doctor that if she couldn't get a good night's sleep, she was determined to kill herself. The doctor mildly replied, "Well, as long as you plan to kill yourself, I suggest you do it by walking yourself to death." The lady did it — and became so exhausted from walking that she collapsed on the bed and fell asleep instant-ly. Exercise makes your body as tired at the end of the day as your mind — and that's a good thing.

And, of course, exercise has a profound effect on your skeletal muscles — those muscles that operate the hinges in your body and allow you to move. When you exercise vigor-ously, these are the muscles that do the work and sustain the most growth.

However, there are two ways that muscles can grow: strength and endurance. Some exercises are designed specifi-cally to make muscles grow larger and more powerful. Weight-lifting is probably the most common exercise of this type. However, this kind of exercise involves tremendous exertions for very short periods of time. The heart doesn't get past the critical threshold value. And while the muscles grow, very little else happens.

The best kind of exercise for overall health is endurance exercise —much easier actions repeated often. It's much easier to run twenty steps than to lift a two-hundred-pound barbell. However, unless you're in top shape, you can't lift

that two-hundred-pound weight very often in succession —
but you can run much, much more than twenty feet. And as
you run, or swim, or play tennis, or play basketball vigorously
for half an hour or an hour, your heartbeat rate rises past the
critical threshold value and all the benefits of exercise come to
your body. Muscle size increases more slowly this way — but
by improving your blood circulation and your stamina over
long periods of time, you increase your endurance to the
point where hours of exercise on end become possible.

If you want both benefits of exercise — larger muscles and
longer endurance — simply combine them, and add weight-
lifting or other anaerobic exercises to your regimen. But the
aerobic exercises, the ones that improve your circulation,
should come first.

You should also be aware that not all sports are good
exercise. Some sports merely require skill, not great strength
or endurance. Golf, for example, almost never gets anyone's
heart beating past the critical threshold value. Archery provides even less exercise, unless you run from the shooting
block to the target several times in rapid succession! And
bowling provides almost no exercise at all.

Sports that provide good exercise are those which force
you into almost constant activity for extended periods of time.
Tennis is a good sport, along with all its permutations, like
handball and racquetball. Basketball — without the time-outs
— is a good exercise; but baseball is not, particularly if you're
playing catcher or if you get walked a lot! Soccer is much
better exercise than football because it stops less often, and
travels from one end of the field to the other more often; and
extended swimming and running are also good exercises.

It's important as you choose the kind of exercise you want
to pursue that you find one that you enjoy. Calisthenics are
deadly dull, and running can be terribly boring if you're
alone, running the same route day after day. Sports that
involve teams are often hard to set up; but if you can find a
regular tennis partner or a good handball opponent, or if you
can find someone who will run with you in competition, so
that the running won't lose its intrigue, then you'll have a

much better chance of enjoying your exercise. And the more you enjoy it, the more likely you are to want to continue.

After all, why exercise alone? You rarely eat alone, if you can avoid it; you don't like going out on the town alone; and if those activities are more enjoyable with company, so is exercise. And if you're worried that the person you exercise with will think you don't have much ability or stamina, choose someone as out of shape as you, and grow together!

It's important that whenever possible, your exercise take place outdoors. This is as much for the psychological benefit as for the physical. We have too many walls around us — we need to learn to feel space. We need to retreat from central heating and air conditioning long enough to remember we live in a world full of beauty; we need to break down ceilings and walls in order to remember the size of the world around us, and to feel ourselves a part of it.

We get too isolated in our houses, cars, and offices. Exercising outdoors breaks down the barriers. We feel more open and more free — and better able to enjoy the time we do have to spend shut off from most of the outside world.

If you're overweight, exercise has an added benefit. While exercise alone isn't likely to be a very satisfactory method of weight reduction, exercise *can* enhance a sensible diet. A good weight-loss diet will actually leave you feeling more energetic and able to exercise — and if you take advantage of those feelings and work out regularly, your body will respond by using incoming nutrients to build new muscles, which will add to your body's tendency during exercise to use up stored energy. Thus your diet will not only cut down on fat — through exercise, you'll be improving overall health and muscle tone at the same time.

"Take it easy and drop dead," said a headline in a 1974 Russian newspaper. Researchers at the Institute of Gerontology at Kiev gave a preliminary report in May of that year on their research into the relationship between a restful life and aging. And the evidence is already quite clear: "ideal conditions" — that is, food and water readily available without any need for physical activity — killed experimental animals much sooner than they should have been expected to die.

Your body needs rest, of course — proper sleep at night is essential to good health. But along with rest, your body needs exercise — good, solid exercise that strains you toward your physical limits. Just as it's good to stretch your mind beyond its capacities, so is it good to stretch your body. And in both cases, that stretching increases the limits of capacity. Your potential, in the long run, has few limits, both mentally and physically. And if you use your body wisely and well, both in the way you feed it and the way you exercise it, the Lord's promise will surely be fulfilled: You'll run and not be weary, walk and not faint.

As Brigham Young pointed out, "Many persons are so constituted, that if you put them in a parlor, keep a good fire for them, furnish them tea, cake, sweetmeats, etc., and nurse them tenderly, soaking their feet, and putting them to bed, they will die in a short time; but throw them into snowbanks, and they will live a great many years."

The snowbank treatment may not be one you hunger for — but to be healthy you do have to tax yourself physically. It's the kind of tax that doesn't take anything away from you — it returns strength and vigor and health far beyond what you might have expected.

10

It Isn't
All in Your Head

The Johnsons of Detroit, Michigan, were a normal Latter-day Saint family, except that one of their sons had a terrible problem with hyperactivity. He couldn't seem to hold still, was constantly provoking or attacking his brothers and sisters and was by and large impossible to live with.

They tried everything. At a doctor's suggestion they gave the boy sedatives — but watching him walk around the house lethargic and apathetic didn't make the parents particularly happy. They followed a psychologist's advice and ignored him — but the boy was not having normal tantrums. Ignored, he simply went on being destructive, and soon had the house — and the family's life — in shambles.

Finally, a doctor who had been experimenting with nutrition made a much simpler, and yet in some ways more drastic, suggestion. "Take the boy off all junks foods. Give him no sugar if you can possibly avoid it. Feed him only on natural foods. Candy is out. Treats are out. Whole wheat is in."

What difference could that possibly make? the parents asked themselves. But since they'd tried everything else, they tried that, too. Being Latter-day Saints, they were ex-

tremely conscious of family unity — and so in order to keep
the hyperactive boy from feeling persecuted, they changed
the entire family's diet, not just his. Sugar was out for every-
body; whole wheat was in.

The results were shocking. The boy almost immediately
stopped his antisocial behavior and became a normal —
though still somewhat rambunctious — child. He slept better.
He found healthier outlets for his creative impulses.

But that wasn't the big surprise. What really shocked the
parents was the difference the new diet made to the rest of the
family. "We hadn't known we had a problem," Sister
Johnson later said. "But all of a sudden we realized that we
were all quarreling less. We were less irritable. We liked each
other better. We had more fun. We felt more like doing
things. We worked harder and got less tired doing it. It was
wonderful."

Of course, once everything was going smoothly, they
began to feel that they could slack off a little. One week they
had sugar products three times — cake, a candy treat, and
some ice cream. "Almost immediately, everything fell apart,"
Sister Johnson reports. "We started getting snappish with
each other. And our little boy started picking on his sisters
again and again being destructive."

So they went back on the diet and things went back to
blissful peace again.

Much of our mental anguish in life is, of course, caused by
disobedience to the Lord's commandments, or by our inability to get along well with other people. However, a large
amount of our irritability, our fears, our neuroses really
doesn't arise in our minds. It starts in our stomachs, with the
way we eat, the way we live.

And it isn't all diet, either. Exercise often has the same
beneficial effect. Parents have known for years, instinctively,
that letting the children wear themselves out running around
in the yard is a good cure for the indoor wiggles. What parents
forget is that they, too, need to wear themselves out in good
physical exercise in order to calm frazzled nerves or soothe
worries. In the old days, if a man got angry with his wife — or
vice versa — he could go outside and chop wood until he felt

better. She could take the laundry to the stream and scrub it out until her back was tired and her heart was at peace.

Nowadays, though, we rarely take advantage of opportunities for physical release of our emotions — and our work no longer forces us to labor physically. There is no clinical proof of this, but I suspect that child abuse and wife abuse and husband abuse may stem from the utter frustration of never having any physical release of tension. Because there's no strenuous physical activity, eventually the penned-up frustrations take themselves out in mad, savage attacks on the very people a person loves most. Child abusers, after all, rarely appear abnormal in their daily lives. It's only in the way they seek physical release of their angers and fears that they differ from the norm.

And scientists are beginning to discover that even schizophrenia may well have a physical cause, a missing enzyme or series of enzymes, which proper diet or exercise may be able to correct, if the enzyme can't be synthesized.

Our mental health is not something separate from our bodies. We are a united system. The Lord told us the spirit and body are the soul of man. We are one being, not two, and just as the spirit can affect the body, so can the body affect the spirit.

Besides helping our mental health in extreme cases, exercise can be a great help in our general feeling of well-being. Friendships begun on the tennis court can last in every other facet of life. Shared experiences of growth and development of the body also help develop mutual respect and appreciation.

Also, if we choose to get our exercise in a sport that requires skill, we soon develop dexterity that can be transferred to many other activities. A mind made alert on the basketball court is a mind that is also alert in the office or caring for the children.

It is no accident that people with severe mental problems usually have severe physical problems, too. I worked for eight years in a mental hospital, and I became convinced that one of the best — perhaps *the* best treatment for a mental problem was physical reconstruction. Good nutrition and plenty of exercise go a long way toward restoring physical and mental equilibrium.

After all, pyschologists have been able to induce neurotic behavior in both rats and people by manipulating their diet — can't neurotic behavior then be helped by manipulating diet in the other direction? Animals kept in close confinement so that they can't exercise quickly become psychotic — can't giving people a lot of exercise help to cure their psychoses?

Other aspects of mental growth are affected by exercise and nutrition. Students learn better when they're properly fed and their bodies are in good condition. Managers are better able to deal with problems and mothers are better able to keep the peace in the family when they have bodies in tip-top physical condition.

I'm pleased to see that Brigham Young University is leading the way as one of the few major universities in the world to take an active interest in the health of its students. Students coming into the university are tested and measured to see how physically fit they are. Those who are overweight are given physical education courses and instruction in diet to help them get into shape. Those who are weak and flabby are given exercise courses to build strength and stamina. Though the project still won't be of much help to students who refuse to make fitness a way of life, it still goes a long way toward realizing the gospel ideal of educating and perfecting the whole soul of a man or woman — body and spirit, matter as well as mind.

However, there are as many quacks offering exercise placebos as there are quacks selling phony medicines and meaningless "health" diets. You should beware of anyone offering an "easy way to health and fitness." There is only one way to health and fitness: proper food and proper exercise. No one gimmick will give that to you.

Magic belts around the waist do little to help you trim your muscles — unless you exercise strenuously, in which case you don't need the belt! Bicycling machines are a lot less fun than riding a bicycle; isometric exercisers are only as valuable as the amount of work you put into using them. In other words, the real value of any exercise or sports device is in the amount of physical work you do — and it's so easy to get good exercise with very little expense that it seems silly to help make someone else rich for supplying you with gimmicks that you just don't need!

Besides, the more money you put into one type of exercise, the less likely you are to get the variety you need to get well-rounded physical development. Swimming is probably the only exercise that can claim to develop the whole body; running doesn't come very close to that goal, and most other exercises are even farther behind. A good mixture of exercise keeps your exercise program interesting — and develops all your muscles, not just the ones required for a particular activity.

In developing your body, you just can't ignore your mind. If you aren't interested in your exercise, you'll eventually tire of it and quit. Likewise, in developing your mind, you can't ignore your body. If you aren't in good physical shape, your brain — which is, after all, a physical organ — just can't function very well.

11

Good Sense on the Playing Field

Let's face it. If even doctors, who usually try to keep up with advances in the field of medicine, aren't aware of many aspects of good nutrition and exercise, athletic coaches are even less likely to know what they're talking about. It isn't all that long ago that coaches were found to be slipping their athletes amphetamines — speed — a devastating drug that allows a player to overwork himself critically. And we're all too familiar with coaches who believed the ridiculous myth that it was bad to drink water during football practice — and so killed several of their players who dehydrated from working out under the hot sun without water.

Latter-day Saint parents would be wise to keep careful watch on what their children who are involved in athletics are eating and what kind of physical workout they're getting.

One of the most important concerns for parents should be the age at which children begin certain sports. Teenagers and preteenagers still have softer bones than adults; the ends of long bones in the arms and legs are still growing, and hard shocks or violent strains can cause permanent crippling damage.

Hardball pitching, for example, before the early teens can permanently ruin a would-be pitcher's arm. The elbow and shoulder never recover from the damage done. And while we hear most about "old football injuries" that leave adults with trick knees, tackle football before the mid-teens can permanently confine young players to wheelchairs.

Competitive sports instill many valuable ideas in young people — the need for teamwork, good sportsmanship, the desirability of excellence. But when those sports begin prematurely, the more violent ones can leave physical and emotional scars that never heal.

And yet there are sports that can be engaged in by children that are relatively safe. Soccer, basketball, and other presumably noncontact sports can be good exercise. And childhood games, like tag, are often better exercise than most adults get — can *you* keep up with your children in a game of tag?

When your children want to enter a serious athletic program in high school, it becomes a different matter. They are usually physically mature enough by mid-teens to begin seriously training for athletic excellence. But the kind of performance they'll be expected to put out requires more than mere physical fitness. They have to be super-fit, able to perform athletic feats far beyond what is required to keep the body functioning normally.

An athlete seeks to do for his body what Einstein and other geniuses did for their minds — hone it until it is a perfect tool that will respond to every demand, no matter how severe, that he can put on it. That requires much more exertion than the half hour or hour a day of exercise most people need.

That's why coaches adopt rigid training courses. Most of them still understand little about nutrition, and require massive intakes of muscle meats, severe weight changes through the use of salt tablets or sweating, and doses of sugar before strenuous contests. Some are beginning to change that regimen to one that actually works better — but most coaches are primarily interested in fielding a winning team. Whatever will benefit the team is all the coach wants, and as far as the athlete's individual needs are concerned, unless he's one of the starring players he has to be ready and able to take care of himself.

As far as physical exercise is concerned, athletes need to be careful to drink a lot of water, particularly during the summer months. During strenuous exercise, the muscles heat up — that energy is released in the form of heat. In order to keep the body from burning up and dying, perspiration is released. The sweat is hot, and as it evaporates it carries off the heat with it.

However, the water that leaves the body during perspiration has to be replaced. Without water, individual cells shrivel and die; blood is harder to pump when there isn't enough water in it; circulation becomes sluggish; and if an athlete doesn't make sure he keeps plenty of water in his system, he can kill himself. If he survives, he'll certainly be sick. Permanent brain damage can result from dehydrating during exercise.

Coaches generally know which exercises will build up athletes in the required ways, but athletes still need to be careful. It wasn't that long ago that a coach punished a player by making him run full tilt into a tackling bag, headfirst, time after time. Finally the player simply fell down. He never got up again — the damage to the spine and brain from the repeated shocks was too much for his nervous system. Avoid direct shocks that follow the line of your backbone — rather absorb shocks with your shoulders.

There is no exercise and no equipment right now to protect a football player's knees — for that reason, it's a good idea to be careful of the kind of pivoting that is done. All the body's joints have limits, and strain beyond those limits will result in injury.

So far as an athlete's diet is concerned, everything that goes for normally healthy nutrition applies to athletes, only more so. An athlete in severe training needs double the normal number of calories — 6,000 — just to maintain his weight. And because of the strains that athletic training puts on the body, cells die faster and must be replaced. However, athletes should remember that they are eating more in order to meet their *energy* requirements. Energy comes best from starches —

the complex carbohydrates — since these digest slowly and evenly, providing the right amount of energy in the bloodstream throughout the day. Protein isn't a good energy food, and so only about 12 percent of the athlete's diet needs to be protein. Any more than that will simply be passed out of the body anyway — putting a great strain on the bowels, the liver, and the kidneys on the way.

The last meal before an athletic competition should be moderate, neither unusually heavy nor unusually light. The last thing an athlete's body needs is to be starving while trying to perform at peak capacity — as soon as the body thinks it isn't being fed enough, it starts conserving energy, and the result is a weakening of athletic performance. Likewise, a huge meal takes a long time to pass through the digestive system, and while the athlete needs all his energy for competition, much of it is being diverted to the digestion of that big meal.

Moderation avoids the two extremes and helps the athlete stay at his peak.

Also, if you have an athlete in your family, you need to make sure that he or she doesn't fall into the habit of "crashing" — getting out of shape during the off-season of a particular sport, and then trying to work back into top condition just in time for the beginning of the season. It's much better to stay in top or near-top condition year-round. A football player should also make sure he has a winter and spring sport, like handball or tennis, to keep up strength and agility. A track and field man needs to make sure he stays in shape even when competition is months away. By staying in shape, an athlete allows himself or herself to start out closer to the desired peak performance — which raises the chances of doing really remarkable things during competition.

And even athletes who want to pursue a career in their sport need to remember this: There isn't a sport in the world that can be played in top form forever. There eventually comes a time when an athlete will have to quit. It only makes sense, then, that the athlete should be certain that his sport has brought him physical fitness, and not a lopsided development that gives him some skills, but no continuing physical activity that he can keep into old age. Football doesn't last past the thirties; a forty-year-old pitcher is rare; basketball players have a very short competitive life. Gold medal winners in the Olympics are rarely in their thirties; champion swimmers are rarely much out of their teens.

That's why an athlete should make sure that he does nothing that will cripple him and keep him from being physically active when his sport is through. And he should make sure that he has a sport that he enjoys that can be played even into old age. Bicycling, running, tennis, and other variable-pace sports can be adjusted to meet the needs of the athlete — an old man can still cycle to his heart's content, though he may be slower than he was in his youth, but few old men can play even decent football. The lifelong sports need to be developed along with the sports of youth, if the value of athletic activity is to be continued. There is nothing sadder than seeing a former football hero in his forties, paunchy, weak, and unhealthy, because he didn't have any other sport he enjoyed when his days of football glory ended.

And that's important — in the competitive team sports it's possible to win a lot of local, temporary fame — and in some cases fame can be national or international. There's nothing wrong with being recognized for excellence, but the parents of the athlete should make sure that he knows from an early age that the real value of sports is in the fun of the game and the joy of being physically fit. Long after the fame is gone — or never came — those rewards go on and on and on.

III

Getting It Together

Good nutritional habits, proper exercise — for total fitness add a positive, wholesome attitude to life and an involvement in purposeful, uplifting activities of body, mind and spirit.

12

You Won't Find Health at the Doctor's Office

When do you go to the doctor? When you're sick, of course. When something is happening to you that you don't understand. When you can't cope with the normal events of your life.

But when everything is fine — or at least not unusually bad — you leave the doctor alone.

Medicine is like any other profession. It is geared toward meeting demand. Doctors learn what they need to know in order to treat patients. And patients usually come to doctors with severe problems. That's where doctors' expertise is, and that's what they should be consulted for.

You wouldn't go to a contemporary corporate lawyer to find out about the laws of inheritance of titles and lands in fourteenth century England — there isn't much demand for that knowledge today, and the lawyer just isn't likely to have it. You wouldn't go to a modern plumber to find out about Roman and Cretan plumbing systems in the centuries before Christ, either — those ideas, while once known, have been forgotten.

Likewise, few doctors have prepared themselves to teach you much about the way you should live to be healthy. They are involved in treatment, not prevention, of disease. They're soldiers in a war against illness and tragedy — but during the peacetime, when you aren't particularly ill, they just don't know what to do.

That's why the Lord's instructions are particularly valuable to us. They are the guidelines that point the way to what we need to do to stay in good health — without ever having to call the doctor. Of course proper nutrition and exercise aren't infallible — some cancers can still strike, hereditary diseases can't be prevented, and influenza can still get you. But your body is better prepared to cope with such emergencies if it is otherwise in perfect health. If your system is rundown, even the best doctor can't make much headway in the war against disease.

However, just because doctors aren't highly trained in the field of nutrition doesn't mean that we can afford to ignore what they say. There are doctors pursuing serious research into nutrition, and for all that science hasn't cured every problem in the modern world, the scientific method is still a good way of finding things out. The Lord doesn't reveal what man's own intelligence can tell him, and it's a foolish man or woman who automatically rejects doctors' advice just because it comes from doctors.

After all, doctors do have to pass through certain courses and examinations — they have to have some grounding in knowledge of the way the human body functions. While they don't have all the answers, it's rare to find a doctor who will deliberately lie or falsify the evidence on a certain question. But because nutrition is an area where doctors just don't know as much as they do about medicine and surgery, the field of nutrition and exercise is one where many quacks operate, preying on the ignorance of people who are looking for answers — particularly easy answers. Nothing is more tragic than people taught by quacks that they shouldn't go to doctors for cancer treatment — when that treatment might have saved their lives. And nothing is more tragic than people spending their money and poisoning their bodies and buying and using "nutritional" or "health" diets, foods, or pills that amount to nothing more or less than patent medicines.

Not long ago I was in Provo, Utah, attending a "free lecture on nutrition." Newspaper advertisements before the event called the lecturer a *doctor* — but he was neither a doctor of medicine nor a doctor of nutrition. In fact, his doctorate was in a field totally unrelated to health and nutrition. When an old man in the audience asked the lecturer why he spent the money to come to Provo and lecture absolutely free, the lecturer answered, "I have a deep concern and respect for nutrition and health."

Sounds altruistic and noble, doesn't it? But in fact, this lecturer was no different from the patent medicine salesmen who used to sell devastating drugs as cures for everything from hangnails to heart disease.

The lecturer had a smattering of nutritional knowledge, and he was clever enough to sound very well-informed. But, unfortunately, all of his information was twenty-five years out of date. He kept stressing that the only good sources of protein were meat, fish, eggs, and milk; that no matter what you eat or how much you eat, you still need vitamin supplements; and just by coincidence, he happened to be associated with a firm that sold those vitamin and mineral supplements that he claimed we so badly needed.

We don't need them.

But many people seem to enjoy sneering at the findings of science. While science has occasionally made some spectacular errors, those errors have always been discovered and eliminated by scientists working carefully to find more truth. And while researchers are still on the threshold of the fascinating field of nutrition, their findings so far are much more firm and much more trustworthy than the prattlings of self-proclaimed experts who sell nutrition ideas that they just made up or that they heard someone else, equally ignorant, preach.

Perhaps the best test of this is that as science has slowly advanced in knowledge, it has time and again reached the ideas that the Lord revealed to his prophets decades and centuries before. Science catches up with revelation — and

Latter-day Saints would be wise to take advantage of the fact that we already have information that scientists have yet to learn!

Eventually, one of the best things that could happen to our society is to have community fitness centers available to every single family in the industrialized nations, where fitness is difficult under ordinary circumstances. Instead of being prey to quacks or out-dated ideas, people could be kept in touch with the latest findings of competent researchers; fads could be replaced by sensible, well-thought-out lifestyles that lead to health and fitness. And such centers would have to be completely nonprofit, with no axe to grind, since "ideologies" and the profit motive often distort people's teachings and mingle falsehood with the truth.

In the meantime — for I doubt such centers will spring up spontaneously in the near future — every family can be its own comprehensive fitness center. The simple principles outlined so far in this book are completely livable by every Latter-day Saint family — in fact, by every family in the country. With a minimum of expense, and relatively costless changes in diet, Latter-day Saint families could easily follow the complete Word of Wisdom, becoming not just healthier than our sick, sick society, but rather absolutely healthy, free of the disease and weakness that come from poor nutrition and a sedentary lifestyle.

Total fitness, of course, is a balance of social, emotional, spiritual, intellectual, and physical activities. A lonely person who can't cope with social situations, who has no friends, and who just isn't happy is unlikely to be able to develop real health and fitness. A person who can't control his emotions, or who has lost all spiritual contact with God, or who never does anything that provides intellectual stimulation just can't be fully happy — and therefore can't be fully healthy. A fine athletic body is no cure for the misery that comes from disobedience and sin; good nutrition and the absence of disease can't compensate for a terrible temper that drives family members into fear or loathing of the person who can't seem to control his emotions.

It is impossible, in other words, to completely cure a person's ills without treating his entire life. We are not a collection of independent attributes. We are complex systems of interrelated events. We are spirits with bodies that live in a world of other spirits with bodies, and how we get along with others, with God, with our own minds, and with our bodies has a cumulative effect.

Stomach aches and ulcers can come from anxiety and worry.

Anger and irritability can come from poor nutrition.

Physical lethargy and weakness can come from loneliness.

Overeating is often a symptom of self-loathing or other emotional problems.

Misery is often a consequence of sin.

A dull mind is often a symptom of a weak, unused, mistreated body.

To be completely happy and healthy, we can't ignore any one aspect of total fitness and total health. That's one of the most exciting things about the gospel of Jesus Christ. The Lord told Joseph Smith that there is no distinction between physical and spiritual things with the Lord — all things are spiritual to him, meaning that every aspect of our lives is a matter of the Lord's concern.

One of the greatest blessings of this knowledge is that Latter-day Saints are able to call upon the Lord in any work they perform. A businessman with difficult decisions, a housewife with problems among the children, a person who is trying to start a new exercise program that will perfect his or her body, or someone seeking to obey the full Word of Wisdom — they can all call upon the Lord for help and counsel.

And the Lord responds. After all, he will only rejoice at anything we do to increase our happiness and the happiness of those around us. "Man is that he might have joy," we've been told, and the Lord's whole purpose is to bring to pass our ennoblement and fulfilment as individuals.

So far as our physical health is concerned, many factors work to decide how healthy we'll be. The first factor, of course, is heredity and environment — the set of circumstances we find ourselves in. Many children are born with birth defects, which they can do little or nothing about — tragically, many of these defects are now being clearly linked with alcohol and tobacco and the use of other drugs. Children of parents who use these things start out with strikes against them, and it's much harder for them to achieve complete health and fitness.

The early environment is something else over which individuals have little control. A child who grows up in a cloud of tobacco smoke can hardly be blamed for being accustomed to the smell — and even for having a physical dependence on it. A child who is overfed in infancy has a much harder time getting rid of excess fat than one who first became obese in adulthood. A malnourished infant can suffer physical and mental damage that is impossible to repair. But at the same time, an infant raised with proper nutrition and good attitudes and experiences in the areas of eating and exercise has a head start toward complete physical health in later years.

As a child grows up, he begins to have more effect on his own physical well-being. These voluntary factors in physical health are exercise, nutrition, and rest. In each area, children need to be taught — and adults need to acquire — good habits.

In nutrition, we need to eat a balanced diet that includes as many of the nutrients the Lord has distributed through the available food supply as possible. Concentrating on one food to the exclusion of all others, or allowing whole types of food to be eliminated, can severely weaken us. Also, the modern practice of stripping whole foods down until few of the original nutrients are left needs to be avoided. If food producers realized that the public actually preferred healthful foods, the profit motive would bring those foods to the marketplace far faster than any legislation possibly could.

Also, harmful substances need to be avoided. As we have seen, commercial sugar is one of the most harmful — and most prevalent — of our self-administered poisons. Overuse of meat is another danger, and we should follow the Lord's advice to eat it sparingly, except when we really need it. And potentially harmful preservatives, additives, and insecticides need to be carefully investigated to see just what effects they will have on our bodies. If you don't know what a chemical is going to do to you, is it really safe to eat it? Many chemicals have no noticeable short-range effects, and only cause harm over a long period of time. (However, one shouldn't be paranoid about "chemicals." After all, every reaction in our body that keeps us alive is a chemical reaction — without chemicals, we'd be dead! We need to avoid *harmful* chemicals, not *all* chemicals.)

Besides nutrition, we need to make sure we get well-balanced exercise. Just any exercise isn't enough — we need to be sure our regular exercise program includes significant aerobic exercise to build up our endurance and our coronary strength. Also, we need to be sure we get a variety of exercise, since one type alone will rarely meet our needs completely.

Exercise should also be a pleasure, not drudgery. Our attitude toward exercise makes a real difference in the value it has for us. If we don't enjoy it, we approach it as an unpleasant duty, and whether we mean to or not, we slacken our efforts. In order to put everything into our exercise, we have to really enjoy it — once again linking the emotional with the physical.

Another requirement for good health and fitness is adequate rest. How much sleep should we get? Enough. And how much is enough? One of the best ways to find out is, after a day with plenty of exercise and proper food, to go to bed early enough that you will automatically wake up at the time you need to rise.

At first, of course, your body habits will wake you up at the normal time, even though the alarm doesn't go off anymore. But over a period of weeks, your body soon gets used to sleeping properly for an entire night, and wakes itself up at the right time.

It's important, however, to get up as soon as you wake up (after a reasonable amount of sleep, of course). If you lie in bed, you'll probably go back to sleep, and oversleeping can be as enervating as overeating. If you are in good health, you will be going to bed tired and sleepy and wakening in the morning feeling completely ready to get up and begin another day.

The right balance of rest, good nutrition, and proper exercise go a long way toward eliminating symptoms we have for too long associated with middle and old age. Too often they are really symptoms of long-term neglect and mistreatment of our bodies, and not the number of birthdays we've had at all.

Good physical health will eliminate many symptoms of aging — or postpone them for years. However, once again our body and spirit together make up a complex system. Even if we're in perfect physical health, if we stop having a sense or feeling of purpose, we tend to age faster; or if we stop using our minds, we tend to become senile more easily. Nutrition, exercise, and rest need to be accompanied by real involvement in family, community, and intellectual activity — and a close relationship with the Lord.

It's important to remember, however, that age *does* come, and with it comes some curtailment of our youthful activities. We will still slow down, however we keep ourselves in good shape. Heredity has a lot to do with this — children of people who lived to a ripe old age are more likely to live that long than children of people who died younger. But despite those limitations — and the knowledge that the Lord intends the curtain to close on our life after a reasonable time — we can make our lives more enjoyable by having good health. I have seen seventy-year-old men and women in better physical shape than men and women in their forties — and the difference was not in one single factor, but rather in many. The prematurely old middle-aged people tended to be overweight, weak, sedentary, poorly nourished, unhappy, irritable, hard to live with. However, the vigorous old people tended to be physically active, properly nourished, cheerful and optimistic, actively involved in the world around them, and trying to live righteous lives, according to whatever creed they believed in.

That's the difference, of course. And Latter-day Saints have everything they need to guide them to long, full, happy, productive lives. If they'll practice the principles that have been taught in the Church for a century and a half already. If they'll step back from their busy lives and take a long, hard look to see just how they're actually treating their bodies and their spirits. If they'll take the trouble to obey!

One important note concerns jogging. This low-level running has become a national fad — to the point that in some communities it's almost an institution. Jogging has become an obsession, and one of the chief things that people think of when they think of exercise and physical fitness. And yet jogging is one of those exercises that actually can cause more harm than good. It would be so much better if some of the time expended in jogging could go toward equally worthy activities that are less harmful, more helpful — and, to be frank, a lot more fun.

Why isn't jogging the best exercise?

1. Jogging only improves muscle tone in the lower portion of the trunk and in the legs. It needs to be accompanied by other exercises in order to build muscle tone elsewhere; whereas swimming, tennis, and many other activities provide much more balanced exercise.

2. Joggers are prone to measure themselves against other joggers — often joggers who've been working at it for some time. Someone who isn't in good physical shape is often likely to overtax himself — and if he already has heart problems, too much jogging too quickly can kill him. Remember! When jogging becomes competitive it is no longer a physical fitness activity, and competitive athletics are only for those already in excellent physical condition.

3. The constant pounding on hard pavement or other running surfaces can cause excessive joint strain in the foot, ankle, knee, hip, sacroiliac, and lumbosacral joints, and also the joints in the spine. Shin splints — strain of the muscles along the shin — also commonly occur to joggers, and there have been many cases of achilles tendon problems. Since there are many exercise programs that don't include these strains, jogging should certainly not be the largest part of your exercise program.

4. Jogging is, bluntly, boring. There's a limit to how many different types of scenery are available within jogging distance of your home. And jogging is utterly lacking in that keen concentration needed in other sports. While jogging can

be competitive, it still doesn't require the kind of competitive edge needed in a good game of tennis or handball, and it doesn't even offer the exhilaration of a sprinting race.

5. Jogging doesn't help you become more flexible. The range of motion of your arms and legs is quite limited — you never really have to stretch very far. Unless you have exercises or other physical activities that provide that stretching, you just aren't getting all the physical development you need.

6. Jogging tends to worsen rather than improve the most common posture problems. While with many sports you're forced to adopt many different positions, in jogging you stay in roughly the same position all the time. It doesn't wake up and strengthen muscles all along your spine or in your shoulders, and in fact is likely to make your posture even worse than it was before. To improve posture, you have to use your body in many different positions, stretching and elongating your muscles.

7. Jogging is so specific — that is, it develops such a limited range of muscles — that even when you are in good shape for jogging, you aren't necessarily in good shape for anything else. Good exercise should prepare you for many different activities, but by and large joggers are able to jog. Period.

I wouldn't have devoted so much space to showing the problems and limitations of jogging if it weren't for the fact that jogging is so much in the public consciousness that when most people think of exercise, they think of getting out in the morning and running a few miles. And this may well be one of the main reasons why so few people actually do start an exercise program. Jogging doesn't appeal to them — and they think that because everyone else is jogging, that's what *they'd* have to do, too.

But there are so many other possibilities for exercise — though jogging could be a *part* of your exercise program — that you can have as varied a diet of physical activity as you'd want to have of food. You couldn't face the same salad day after day, week after week — so why condemn yourself to jogging away, slopping your body along the same boring pavement again and again?

Latter-day Saints are in a better position than any other people on earth to testify that the Lord loves and cares for all of his children. He is concerned about every aspect of our lives; he wants us to be joyful. And because he loves us, he's given us guidelines for treating each other, for dealing with him, for building our families, for resisting temptation, for enriching our minds — and for building our bodies into the beautiful, well-running tabernacles he meant them to be.

Isn't it time to follow the Word of Wisdom — the whole revelation, and not just the specific commandments required of us for temple attendance? If we love the Lord, we keep his commandments — and every word of advice he offers to us.

It doesn't cost much. And what we get in return is happiness, the pleasure of feeling good, and a greater capacity for enjoyment of life.

"And all saints who remember to keep and do these sayings, walking in obedience to the commandments, shall receive health in their navel and marrow to their bones;

"And shall find wisdom and great treasures of knowledge, even hidden treasures;

"And shall run and not be weary, and shall walk and not faint.

"And I, the Lord, give unto them a promise, that the destroying angel shall pass by them, as the children of Israel, and not slay them. Amen." (D&C 98:18-21.)

The advertisers of junk foods promise a lot of things.

But they can't match the promise the Lord offers the Saints who take his advice.

And the best thing about the Lord's promises is that he keeps them. The Word of Wisdom really works. It will work for you.

Appendix

PRINCIPLES OF PHYSICAL FITNESS

1. Everyone enjoys some level of physical fitness (whether it be high or low), and it is constantly changing. Above-normal levels of activity will improve fitness levels, while sedentary living will allow you to be just like most of your friends.

2. It took longer than three or four weeks to establish your present level of physical fitness and it is going to take longer than a few weeks to make worthwhile changes.

3. Instant programs of fitness and weight reduction merely help you to think that you have attained a goal you have not yet reached.

4. Being physically fit does not require that you train for the Olympics. Three exercise sessions a week of about thirty minutes' duration are sufficient to build and maintain a

fairly high level of fitness. No one is too busy to fit that much time into his busy lifestyle!

5. There is no magic about the time of day you exercise or the types of exercises you do. The magic is all in the fact that you exercise consistently over a long period of time.

6. The system has a natural tendency to return to previously established and accepted (accepted as "normal") levels of ability.

7. Muscular functions are interrelated to such a degree that it is almost impossible to isolate the function of one particular muscle.

8. Sudden movements against resistance are the most dangerous types of movements — and the degree of the resistance is usually of less importance. Stretching exercises intended to increase range of motion should not be quick, jerky movements.

9. Do not make any attempt to compare yourself with any other individual — unless you happen to have an identical twin, and even then there are some physical differences. Far too many factors are involved for a rational comparison between individuals.

10. Moderation is a good rule to follow in exercise as well as in eating. Exercise sessions should begin with a warm-up period and end with a cooling-down phase. It is far better to progress slowly into exercise and fitness than to have to nurse injuries in the form of pulled muscles, tendons and ligaments. You should always end an exercise session feeling that you could easily do more.

11. Fat deposits are an overall situation, with naturally heavier concentrations in some parts of the body. (A certain amount of fatty tissue is equally as normal as average levels of muscular size and strength.)

12. The addition of fat is a result of a positive calorie balance (eating more than you require); reduction of fat is produced by a negative calorie balance (burning more energy than you take in in food).

13. "Spot reduction" of fatty tissue is an *outright myth* — a physical impossibility. You can get rid of fat in the abdominal area by the identical method you would use to reduce it in any other area of the body by simply reducing your intake of food, or by increasing the amount of overall exercises, or both. You cannot do it by increasing the amount of abdominal exercise. In effect — and *in fact* — you can reduce fatty tissue in the area of the waist by working your legs (or your arms, or your shoulders, or any other muscle group in your body). It is not necessary to work the midsection in order to reduce fat in the midsection. And absolutely nothing in the way of an artificial aid will do anything to help reduce girth. All that matters is overall consumption of calories; energy output in relation to food input.

14. Much of the weight loss on a semistarvation diet is quickly regained, because a large part of the weight loss is not fatty tissue but lean muscle mass and water. This is rapidly replaced when eating is resumed.

15. It is relatively easy to lose pounds on any low-calorie diet, but after weight loss the dieter goes back to his regular way of eating and regains the weight he has lost — and then some. This is the typical system that most Americans use, the "Yo-Yo" system of girth control.

16. Being overweight and in poor physical condition usually results from the combination effect of four causes:
    1. Too little activity
    2. Too much food
    3. The wrong kinds of activity
    4. The wrong kinds of food
    Trying to correct the problem without giving proper

emphasis to all four of these dimensions is to invite failure and frustration.

When you begin an exercise program, remember that, like most of your friends, you are probably not as physically fit as you think you are, so begin at a level that is sensible for you and progress slowly.

Index